From Bump to Grind

The Secret Scoop on Labor, Delivery & Early Motherhood

SARAH WORKMAN CHECCONE

DEDICATION

For Mark

TABLE OF CONTENTS

ACKNOWLEDGEMENTS

Thank you to the many PPSF mothers, volunteer SISTERs, and friends who have generously shared their stories to help new mothers everywhere. Through your honesty and vision you have allowed your perinatal experiences—though difficult or even heartbreaking—to be purposeful and relatable to benefit countless women and their families. With my whole heart, I thank you.

FOREWORD

This book was written for you, Mama. To reduce your stress as you adjust to motherhood, ease your birth/postpartum transition and put some peer support in the palm of your hand. Literally. After all, moms weren't meant to do this alone.

If you are pregnant or have a baby under 12 months, you are in the "Perinatal Period," and likely in the midst of the most significant life transition you'll ever experience. A lot goes down in those 21 months from conception to baby's first birthday, including many things we never, ever expected.

When we, as moms-to-be, prepare to bring baby home, we have certain dreams and expectations. We buy things, read books, take classes, and politely nod (usually) as advice and anecdotes are heaped upon us. We focus on making it through pregnancy and giving birth, and imagine our maternal instincts will take over when our little cutie is in our arms. Preparing for baby is so important, both logistically and psychologically, but there's another new person coming home after delivery, too. A new mother.

As new (postpartum) mothers, our wellness is crucial to the whole new-baby operation getting off the ground, and if we have to juggle taking care of a newborn *while* trying to figure out the unexpected physical and mental complexities of birth and postpartum, it's just too much. This extra processing requires additional emotional energy and adds postpartum stress to an already exhausted new mom's plate—right when she needs to focus on her own and her baby's wellness. The more I speak with new mothers, the more I am certain a lack of open, honest communication about birth and the postpartum process is seriously counterproductive– even dangerous–to maternal and infant health.

If women in the perinatal period have real information about birth and postpartum-related issues that could and commonly do arise (though they are rarely discussed), they can reduce their postpartum stress and lessen their risk for Postpartum Distress (Depression, Anxiety, etc.). No one can be prepared for every scenario, but what if a new mom could "expect the unexpected" to some degree? For example, what if a new mom could know...

- Many new mothers have stressful hospital stays
- A lot of women don't feel the immediate bond with their babies that they expected
- A majority of new moms feel frustrated and angry that their own lives have changed much more than their partners'
- It's common for a new mom to feel a loss of her own identity and really miss her old self and her old freedom in the first year of motherhood

If she knew these truths and more, maybe she wouldn't feel as afraid, alone, or experience a sense of failure when motherhood isn't quite (or at all) what she expected. Perhaps, she'd feel more comfortable reaching out to someone for support. Real stories help to "normalize the abnormal," and when the going gets tough, that window to reality can be a light in a new mother's darkness.

The miracle of sharing real stories and experiences with other new moms is the "normalizing of the abnormal" (to a reasonable degree–not explaining away the harmful or dysfunctional). When postpartum women get together with other new moms, listen and share their realities, they understand they are not alone in their challenges. Suddenly, a mom in distress doesn't feel like such a "failure" or a "bad mother" anymore. She's just a real mother, with ups and downs like anyone else, doing the best she can.

No matter what you experience as a new mother, please know *you are not alone.* Maybe knowing that is enough for you to deal with the rough stuff and move on, but when the chips are down, face-to-face connection with other women who can relate can be incredibly valuable. Wherever you are, we can help you find the support you want. Email sarahpostpartumfl@gmail.com, call 941.301.8819 or visit www.postpartumflorida.org for more information. Lastly, if you have a story or topic you wish someone had told you before birth, please email me so we can continue to inform and prepare new moms for the crazy postpartum year.

In our Postpartum Support Group, we frequently discuss what we wish we'd known before we gave birth. Then, one day, a group member said to me, "You should write a book about all this stuff–it could really help some new moms." I had to laugh, because that's exactly what I was doing. There's a clear connection between shock and distress. The information in this book aims to lessen some of the shocks of the peak of the perinatal period in order to reduce your stress and distress. And to give you a good laugh, too. Enjoy, and all the best to you, your partner and your baby!

CHAPTER 1

BEFORE BIRTH

Congratulations on your pregnancy and, if you've already given birth, congratulations on bringing your baby into the world! If you've already delivered, please feel free to skip ahead, but you may want to double back and relive and attempt to sort out your birth experience.

You've probably read/are reading other baby and birth books, so we'll skip the typical stuff, i.e., the "birth plan," freezing meals ahead of time and Chapstick in the delivery room. This book is about what *really* happens in labor, delivery and the adjustment of the postpartum year (and how to be prepared for it!). With that in mind, let's start with every pregnant lady's favorite topic... snacks.

Snacks Snacks Everywhere

Pepper your world with diapers and wipes, and also with one-handed, healthier snacks and bottles of water... sometimes getting to the kitchen will be a bridge too far.

As you're nesting, this may be a good time to sprinkle diapers and wipes everywhere–stroller, cars, every bathroom, every floor, etc.– and also one-handed, healthier snacks and bottles of water in every pocket and drawer–the glider, changing table, end tables, nightstands, diaper bag, stroller, bathroom drawers and any and all car consoles.

The freezer/microwave-ready meals are great when you have to feed people other than yourself, but easy, one-handed snacks are the way to go for the first few months. A lot of new moms are surprised that most of their days (and nights) with newborns will be about frequent quality snacking, not meals. Further, they wish someone had told them ahead of time not to keep all the food in the kitchen.

Why? Because in the first three to six months of being a mom, you will frequently be "chairified" (Def: Verb meaning frozen to your chair while trying to get a baby to feed), and nearing light-headed starvation. Getting to the kitchen may simply be a bridge too far. You've got to keep up your own strength, and going without food and water is not going to work. Nutrition and hydration are basic needs, not a "treat" for when our work is done. (P.S., As a mother your work is never "done," just paused until the next round.)

Whether breastfeeding or bottle-feeding, the vigilance and dedication it takes to nurture and nourish a newborn baby is intense. All new moms need to maintain their blood sugar and hydrate like crazy to keep up their strength and mood.

One third-time mom put it simply:

"You don't get any medals for gnawing your arm off while constantly feeding, changing, rocking, and swaying with a baby. You've got to take care of you, and that includes food and water!" – Tracey B.

Perineal Massage & Episiotomy

Episiotomies used to be standard practice, but more and more female OBs are coming out against episiotomies and opting to allow minor tearing instead. You can talk to your doctor about this so you're on the same page before you're chatting through stirrups.

If planning a vaginal birth, talk to your OB or midwife about perineal massage to help prevent an episiotomy. An episiotomy is a minor procedure in which the tissue and muscle between the vagina and the anus is cut to allow for birth, then stitched back together.

I've got to be honest with you, recovery from an episiotomy can be pretty painful. If you have to have one, then so be it. You will heal and be fine. However, please know that this is a topic you can discuss with your provider. Episiotomies used to be standard practice, but more and more female OBs are coming out against episiotomies and instead opting to allow minor tearing of the perineum during delivery.

One OB convinced me of the drawbacks of episiotomy by holding up a piece of paper and gently tugging at opposite corners. "See how it stretches and strains but doesn't tear?" she asked. Then she cut a snip in the center edge of the paper. "Now look what happens…," she said, and tugged again. This time, because of the cut, it tore right down the middle. Message received.

My first delivery resulted in a fourth-degree episiotomy that seriously complicated my recovery, both physically and emotionally. My OB for my second, third and fourth pregnancies was against episiotomies, so we planned to allow some minor tearing during delivery instead. In all three instances, the tearing I experienced resulted in one or two stitches and the pain and recovery were minimal.

Frequently, a small, natural tear is enough to permit vaginal delivery without, as one mom of two put it, *"being opened up like a garage door."* The truth is an episiotomy may be a moment of convenience during birth, but it usually means 7 to 10 days of additional pain for a new mom during her postpartum recovery when she's already dealing with breastfeeding pain, afterpains and everybody's-a-pain pains. If this is important to you, talk with your provider. And if you're having a communication problem, feel free to give him/her my email: sarahpostpartumfl@gmail.com. We'll have a nice long chat.

A Delivery Room Interpreter

A lack of communication in the delivery room, especially under urgent or emergency circumstances, can leave the birthing woman with... the perception of being in danger. This can lead to partial or full Post-Traumatic Stress Disorder following birth.

Most OB appointments are so routine that it can be hard for a pregnant woman to imagine how hectic a delivery room can become. Sometimes things turn urgent, and the parents-to-be may find themselves mentally racing to grasp the complexity of dramatic circumstances.

A breakdown of communication in the delivery room, especially under urgent or emergency circumstances, can leave the birthing woman with feelings of fear, powerlessness, loss of control and the perception of being in danger, which may lead to partial (more frequently) or full Post-Traumatic Stress Disorder (PTSD) following birth. PTSD, partial or full, is a risk factor for Postpartum Distress, including depression and anxiety.

Feeling overwhelmed in the delivery room is not unusual for parents-to-be. Having someone you can trust to explain, interpret and advocate for you can make a world of difference in your comfort level, experience and the memories of your child's birth. Birth doulas are becoming more common in the U.S. as more pregnant women and their partners recognize the value–perhaps the necessity–of having a trained birth support person to guide them through the delivery process.

Expectations & Reality

Some of the new moms in our Postpartum Support Group were shocked to find themselves working through feelings of failure when their births did not go according to their plans.

When we face new experiences we have certain beliefs and expectations. Some people prefer to plan and prepare in order to feel a sense of comfort and control. When it comes to labor and delivery, it can pretty much happen with or without you, and many moms, though they strive to make peace with the unknown, are shocked during labor to realize they may have limited, little or no control over the events of their babies' births. For some women, the challenge is *how the loss of control may make them feel.* There's a wide chasm between knowing something in your mind, and feeling the impact in your heart.

Why discuss this? Because unreasonable expectations about labor, birth and/or motherhood can lead to increased postpartum stress and/or distress. Some of the moms in our Postpartum Support Group were unpleasantly surprised by the disappointment, feelings of failure and other negative emotional aftershocks they experienced when their labors, deliveries and/or postpartum adjustments (early motherhoods) departed from their expectations.

Time after time, new moms have confided that they wished someone had told them *actual* birth and postpartum recovery are far different from one's prenatal fantasies, and that it's healthy to keep your expectations low. I'm not saying it's smart to expect a disaster, only saying it may be wise to set one's goals at basic survival. Anything beyond that is frosting on top.

Birth and bringing home baby are marketed as bliss for commercial purposes only. Modern mythology at work.

I don't bring this up to worry you. If anything, you can feel more confident because you now know perinatal preparation has it's limits. Whatever ends up happening during your delivery and soon afterward, know that while you can't anticipate every issue, you can (and will) recover. Some women find relief and comfort in telling their birth stories (writing about them, talking about them, making memory books–sometimes it's too hard to talk about them/this is not pressure to be crafty) in order to process the complex feelings and sensations of birth, both positive and negative, and find peace.

So, do whatever you prefer to make yourself more comfortable as you look ahead to labor, birth and recovery. Take classes, read books, tour the hospital, interrogate your doctor and pack your hospital bag to the nines. And, as you painstakingly amass duplicates of all your charging cables and tubes of Chapstick like the books and articles advise, you may want to ask yourself questions like, "Can I accept that childbearing is an individual process and that my feelings about my baby's birth may be complicated?" Listen to your answers, or your hesitation or refusal to answer–you may discover some interesting information about yourself. After all, you know you better than anyone else, and open, honest communication with your inner self is going to be really important as you tumble into motherhood.

Constipation and Preparing for Birth

Many new moms say they wish someone had told them that getting their "bathroom ducks in a row" before birth is as important as anything a woman can do to prepare for labor and delivery.

Ah, bathroom matters–a personal, yet vitally important health issue. Both your digestive system and your baby's are going to be at the top of your list for a while. Many women deal with pregnancy constipation, but are unable to imagine how much trouble a sore bum and backed-up bowels can be until the indisposed moment of truth arrives.

Many new moms say they wish someone had told them post-birth bathroom encounters can be really rough for about one to six weeks postpartum, depending on the level of trauma to the perineum during delivery. They further wish their OBs had told them that getting their "bathroom ducks in a row" (that is, achieving regularity) prior to birth would be as important as anything they can do to prepare for childbirth and recovery.

One second-time mom shared her experience:

"I was so mercilessly constipated after my first was born that I swear I needed an epidural just to go to the bathroom. Seriously, in those first few days my bottom was so sore from pushing, I couldn't sit on the couch much less on the toilet. I finally ended up "going" in the shower. It was demoralizing as a first-time mom to go from pregnant goddess to literally standing in my own sh*t in a matter of days, and it definitely made my birth recovery more painful and stressful. I vowed that if I ever had another baby I would not endure that mess again.

When I neared my due date the second time around, I started a high-fiber, lower-sugar ritual-type diet at 32 weeks, and presto—no more constipation. In fact, by the time I delivered, I was doing so well that I was able to 'go' no problem less than six hours post-birth. My nurse was blown away. As a result, my recovery was a hundred times better. What a relief." —Natalie K.

CHAPTER 2

LABOR

Contractions

This part of the birth experience gets the most press, so just a quick mention. A few new moms were surprised that their contractions didn't feel as painful as they had expected and they were able to sleep through a good portion of labor. Other women were disarmed by how horrendous their contractions were. Yet, all new moms in our Group agreed the biggest surprise of the labor process was feeling their bodies take over and operate without permission of their minds.

No Contractions

Some women who delivered by scheduled C-section wished they had known how different the arcs of their birth experiences would be by *not* having contractions. As one first-time C-section mom put it:

"I felt like I missed out on the build-up of labor. There was no process for me. It was like I walked into the operating room and picked out a baby like you pick out bath towels. I was shocked how the lack of labor and vaginal delivery affected me. It seemed to make it harder for me to bond with my baby the first week or so. I just couldn't believe he was the one that was in me for nine months. The whole thing was so surreal."
– Michelle N.

Not all women who have C-sections feel this sense of shock or loss, of course. One's own experience depends on a spectrum of factors. Still, more C-section mamas than I expected expressed some sense of loss over a lack of labor.

Other C-section moms had the… joy? of experiencing hours or even days of contractions before they delivered their babies by caesarean. In those cases, some moms said they felt cheated out of the vaginal deliveries for which they'd labored so arduously, and found themselves needing to work through feelings of loss and disappointment about their cesarean births, too.

Getting Admitted

"I still don't know what happened the first time I was triaged with my oldest, but that cervical check... ugh."

When you are (mostly) sure you are experiencing labor and you go to your hospital or birthing center, it is likely you will first check in at the reception desk. Eventually, a nurse will take you to an examining room to ask about your symptoms and determine whether you are actually in labor. Alternatively, you may be triaged in a cubicle-like setting. Or it may be a combination of the two.

The nurse will ask about your contractions—how far apart are they? How regular are they? How intense are they? She will likely hook you up to a monitor that creates a printout of the frequency, regularity and intensity of the contractions. She also will probably check your cervix to see how dilated (open) and effaced (thinned out) it is, because the more open and thinned out the cervix, the more likely you are in "actual labor" (as opposed to false labor, a.k.a. Braxton-Hicks contractions).

I still don't know what happened the first time I was triaged with my oldest, but I was shocked by that cervical check. Holy moly. No other cervical check had ever hurt that much. I was told later it was because my cervix was still so posterior (pointing back—a sign that you aren't in true labor/haven't progressed much) that the nurse "had to" sort of grab it and pull it down to measure my dilation and effacement. Another first-time mom unfortunately had a similar experience with her first birth:

"She said she was just going to check my cervix. No big deal. I'd been checked every week for the last two months at my doctor's. I scooted down the table, she snapped on a glove and wham! If I'd been closer to the window, I'd have tried to jump out hoping to land on my head. I'd already been laboring for four hours, but the contractions were nothing compared to that." —Kelley H.

Another mom, Gracie W., had quite an experience when she arrived in triage with her first delivery:

"I was the only one in triage when I walked in. The nurse had rushed out to get a patient back to a room before she delivered in the hallway. Then another first-time mom-to-be came in looking just as nervous as I was, but she only spoke Spanish, so we mostly just gestured 'good luck' to each other. Then, a third laboring mom staggered in and dropped to a chair. She kept muttering to herself, hunched in her seat holding her belly. She said something about this being number eight, and just as I was about to ask if she needed the nurse, she clutched her belly and let out a blood-curdling scream that truly stood my hair on end! As she came down from the intensity of the contraction (and the screaming) and began to hunch again, she grunted, took a breath and let out another scream. Every minute. For almost 10 minutes. That is a long time when you are a first-time mom scared out of your wits.

Finally, the triage nurse came back and opened with, 'Okay, who's next?' Immediately both of us pointed in her direction (there was no way to be heard over the screaming). She had her baby less than five minutes later in the hallway en route to L&D. It was enough to make me want to cross my legs and go home."
—Gracie W.

One more thing about getting admitted: Many women feel overwhelmed by busy healthcare settings and think they should "speak only when spoken to." Yet, nurses are only human and may forget to ask you some important questions. If you have news, feel free to lead the conversation.

For example, when I was triaged for my first birth, I knew I was in labor because my water had broken at 5:30 that morning. When the nurse asked about my contractions I responded honestly that they were 5-7 minutes apart. She told me to "go home until they're three minutes apart," due to a bed shortage. Then I suddenly remembered to mention my water had broken.

"Why didn't you say that?" the nurse asked, exasperated because she had to find an empty bed for me. After a painful, soggy drive to the hospital, a circuitous, crampy walk to the floor, then 10 minutes of mayhem in the waiting room followed by 15 minutes of attitude, I was over it. "You didn't ask," I said, exhausted. She frowned and replied thoughtfully, "No, I guess I didn't."

Epidurals

It's easier to get the epidural in place before your labor ramps up because once contractions start coming every 60 seconds you may shake constantly and uncontrollably. Not the best time to aim needles at the old spine.

A few things new moms wish they'd known about epidurals: Getting an epidural does hurt, but hurts far less than a drug-free labor and delivery from what I understand and have experienced. If it's a routine epidural, there should only be a few minutes of pain while the nurse anesthetist or anesthesiologist inserts the needle and the spinal catheter (there is another catheter called a "Foley" or urinary catheter you'll become acquainted with, but first thing's first) in your back. Some women have to have more than one needle stick, so obviously with each needle stick you're, unfortunately, going to have more pain.

It can also be a strange feeling to have your legs go numb, and sometimes one leg loses feeling before the other. Also, once you have the epidural you will be too numb to get up to use the bathroom, hence the urinary catheter. Some women were surprised to learn that having an epidural meant being glued to their beds until after delivery.

It is easier to get the epidural in place before your labor ramps up because once contractions start coming every 60 seconds you may shake constantly and uncontrollably. Not the best time to aim needles at the old spine.

Also, if you get to full or near full dilation, your OB will no longer permit an epidural because you'll be too close to pushing. You need to be able to feel the pressure of the baby in order to push successfully and deliver. So, if you are planning to have an epidural, keep in good communication with your L&D nurse and don't wait too long or you may find the window has closed.

(Quick sidebar–this is not a commercial for birthing with epidurals or in hospitals. Many women have beautiful, drug-free births in hospitals or birthing centers. I bring all this up only because over my five pregnancies, four births and eight years as a mother, I've observed that pregnant women frequently oscillate between denial and terror when it comes to preparing for labor and delivery. Often, they have questions about pain control such as epidurals, but aren't sure whom to ask or how. I aim only to address these unasked or inadequately answered questions in order to reduce your perinatal stress. And give you more to Google.)

Lastly, if you get an epidural, the anesthesiologist or nurse anesthetist may say, "At first you'll feel nothing, then you'll start to feel the contractions again, but just pressure–no pain." Fantastic. However, if you do start to feel the *pain* of the contraction, let your nurse, husband/partner, doula or other birth support person know the medication is not protecting you from pain. Ask for the anesthesiologist or nurse anesthetist as soon as possible and explain what you are feeling so s/he can adjust your dosage prior to birth. If you don't tell the doctor the epidural is no longer working, you could end up fully dilated and needing to push without the pain medication you were counting on. Surprises can be fun, but you don't want that one.

By the way, if you are counting on an epidural for pain control and then on delivery day that option is suddenly off the table, know that this sometimes happens and you will be all right. Take a minute to freak out if need be, but you can have confidence in yourself. You will get through it.

IVs and Catheters

If you deliver in a hospital, you'll most likely have an IV. The medical team taking care of you needs IV access to administer fluids, medication and other necessities directly into your bloodstream in an instant. I imagine some women object, but an IV is part of most hospitals' standard delivery protocol. If you have any questions about this, definitely ask your provider.

The IV needle is usually inserted into a vein on the back of your non-dominant (non-writing) hand. Putting it in hurts more than a blood draw, but it's somewhat similar, and your hand may be mildly sore at the site for 24 hours or so. It's just one of those things. Also, you have to have a urinary catheter if you elect to have an epidural, but they don't put it in until you're numb so it's all smooth sailing.

Maternal & Fetal Monitors

If you just shifted positions and you hear the 'beeeeeeeeep,' there's no need to worry. You probably accidentally moved the monitor off-site. The nurses will come right in and fix it. No sweat.

You may or may not have expected to be monitored during your labor, but if you're in a hospital as opposed to a birthing center, the medical staff will very likely want two monitors on you—one to record and measure your contractions and one to record and measure the baby's heartbeat.

Both monitors are usually round plastic disks, about 3-4" in diameter (like headphones from the '80s), threaded onto wide elastic bands and strapped around your belly. The monitors aren't painful, but they can start to dig into your skin a bit if you sit or turn one way or another for too long.

If you do switch positions and one or more of the monitors get shifted out of place, you'll have the fun of hearing the "beeeeeeeeeep," and seeing your nurse (and possibly others, as well) very purposefully enter your room. Not a big deal—you probably accidentally moved the monitor off-site. The nurse will quickly and easily reposition it.

Dilating

Most first-time moms agree they could not feel their cervixes dilating. Some said they felt the baby "engaging," felt the contractions and, of course, felt the urge to push. But feeling the cervix stretch from zero to 10 centimeters? No. However, I have met women who said they could tell when their cervix was open, but could not pinpoint by how much.

Sometimes women feel disappointed or even foolish because they contract and contract and believe they're progressing when they're actually not. It can be a frustrating stage of the labor process.

Why are we talking about this? Well, because there's a whole population of moms-to-be who labor and walk and squat and roll on birthing balls until you could mistake them for hedgehogs, and after 12-24 hours they're still only dilated about three or four centimeters. *Argh!* And during all that labor they *thought* they *were* progressing/the cervix was opening. It can be very discouraging to work so hard, labor so long and have nothing to show for it.

If this "cervix confusion" happens to you, please know that you are not alone, you're not "out of touch with your body," or "failing at labor," or anything else. The stages and progression of birth can be complex and unpredictable. If what you're doing isn't working, you can talk with your birth/medical team (or look within yourself, if you prefer) and try something else. You will get there. And you are doing great.

Induction & Pitocin

Perinatal research generally goes against elective induction before 39 weeks (visit www.marchofdimes.com for more on this), but well-timed induction past 39 weeks can be a life-saver and has become common practice. Speaking from experience, I was induced with my fourth at 39 weeks after more than a month of non-productive, partially debilitating, wholly annoying contractions which had me on the verge of losing my mind.

It was 109 degrees Fahrenheit the day I went to my final, somewhat-tearful, OB appointment. Upon exam I was cheerfully informed I was "still at a loose 2 (centimeters), Mrs. Checcone!" I could not believe it. Shocked and disappointed, I forced a smile, gave a thumbs-up to the nurse practitioner and turned away before she could see me break down.

After a few minutes, my OB came in and mercifully asked if I would be willing to consider induction. I think she feared that if I went on that way for another 2-3 weeks, caring for three little children in a dangerous heat wave, I might actually burst into flame. "What would you do?" I asked, choking back exasperated tears. "Well, since you're term, I'd go ahead with an induction," she said. "Okaayaayayaayay," I said, breaking into relieved, pregnant sobs.

The induction went beautifully, and I wouldn't change a thing. It did, however, reacquaint me with an old pal of mine from my three previous births–Pitocin.

Induction + vaginal birth (usually) = Pitocin. Many women have shared that they were not mentally ready for the effects of Pitocin, and how rapidly this synthetic version of the natural labor-inducing hormone oxytocin can kick in and accelerate the intensity and frequency of contractions.

Contractions can cause women to shiver and shake, and Pitocin makes for such intense contractions that holding still for the epidural needle post-Pitocin can be more difficult. If you're considering getting an epidural, and the medical team begins talking about starting Pitocin, feel free to raise your hand and ask for that epidural right away before they begin the Pitocin drip.

Pitocin can come on a bit strong, and the nurse may need to dial down the dosage a little until she finds a good level for the baby. Furthermore, while Pitocin can be great for moving things along, it does not always have the desired effect–namely, progression of labor and dilation. This can be tough to take. Repeated changes to the delivery plan, or assurances that a certain approach will work only to have it fail, can feel exhausting to a laboring mom-to-be. Stay strong, Mama. You are still doing great.

Nausea & Vomiting

Ah, the fun of nausea and vomiting in pregnancy seems to never end! Yes, you, too, may have the delight of feeling nauseated and vomiting while in labor. Some women seem to have a reaction to the medication (epidural), some seem to have a reaction to the pain (contractions) and others seem to have just gotten really good at it (that was humor). Seriously, for some moms, acid reflux may be so intense that by the ninth month, presto!! They can randomly vomit before your very eyes!

So how to cope with this unpleasant reality... hmmm... well, at least you're in the hospital so you won't have to clean it up for once, right? And the nurses are quick as a flash with the pans and chucks (the big paper towel-ish things they use to wipe up messes in L&D). That doesn't make it any more pleasant for you, but at least now you know, and if by chance you make it through your last day of this pregnancy without puking... what a bonus.

CHAPTER 3

DELIVERY

Pushing

What is the number one thing moms who give birth vaginally wish someone had told them about pushing? To *pace* themselves, for Lord's sake–don't be a hero! Many moms have confessed they felt some psychological pressure to "impress" their husbands, partners, doctors, doulas, etc., and have some award-winning delivery. Oh, ladies… why do we do this to ourselves?

There is no medal for Competitive Speed-Pushing, my friends. Rudimentary, standard, well-timed pushing is more than sufficient. As long as you trust the folks in the room, just push when you're supposed to and please, *please* consider resting your legs when they tell you to.

I thought the point of pushing was to get the baby out as quickly as possible. Wrong. It can be a very sore surprise that pushing too much too soon and refusing to take the recommended breaks can cause you to pull, strain or tear something you're going to need later. Like your hamstrings.

Too much pushing too fast can cause pulled muscles, especially if you have an epidural because the drugs prevent you from feeling pain (like going to the gym on painkillers = very bad). I was so excited to meet my first baby, I ended up pulling both my hamstrings from having my knees beside my ears for two hours.

After that delivery I couldn't sit down. For days. I couldn't sit in the bathroom, couldn't sit to nurse, couldn't sit in the car going home and couldn't raise my leg to climb a stair. That first night back home, I actually crawled up the front steps of our house like a dog. A brilliant moment in early motherhood.

More On Nausea & Vomiting

Whether it's the drugs or the trauma or just the same marvelous nausea you've been enduring for the past nine months, some women experience nausea and vomiting during delivery, too. It's no fun, but usually you're so focused on getting baby out (and you've probably already thrown up so many times in the last 40 weeks) it's pretty low on your list of concerns.

What may seem vile and repulsive to you is nothing to your nurses. Might as well be an overturned cup of coffee for all the they care.

Labor & Delivery nurses seem to have lightning reflexes when it comes to vomiting and worse (yes, the rumors are true–there is worse). What's more, unless they're super new, *they have seen it all* and nothing fazes them in the slightest. What may seem vile and repulsive to you is nothing to your nurses. Might as well be an overturned cup of coffee for all they care.

Regarding the aforementioned rumors, it is true that pushing baby out means pushing *everything* out. One new mom said:

"I was really excited to watch my baby's birth in the mirror... that is, until I saw that with every push the nurse was having to wipe me. I was pushing out poop with every contraction and I couldn't even feel it (because of the epidural)!! That was the end of the mirror for me, and I was so embarrassed, I missed a contraction. I had heard that some women do that, but I didn't think I was. I am in healthcare myself, so I know the nurses didn't mind, and my husband didn't seem to notice, but, oh my goodness... blecch."–Casey E.

The truth is childbirth is not all triumphant pushing and tears of joy. Some things are going to be disgusting, surprising and overwhelming, and several moms have said they wished they'd known the normal Range of Disgusting for Birth so they didn't spend precious mental energy on embarrassment during labor and delivery. Please know you can be proud of whatever revolting disaster you experience, and claim it as part of *your baby's birth story.* Or live in denial and rapidly develop amnesia. Your call.

Getting Baby Out

It's often quite a surprise to laboring moms-to-be when they take that breath, hold it, push and immediately break all the blood vessels in their faces.

When you're fully dilated you will feel the urge to push, or "bear down" like you're having a bowel movement. If you have an epidural, you will feel only pressure, not pain, way down in your abdomen and pelvis. The nurse will tell you to take a deep breath, hold it and push as if you were, in fact, having a bowel movement. She may even put her fingers at the entry to the vagina and tell you to push her fingers out. Weird and gross, perhaps, but most say the technique helps.

It can be quite a surprise to laboring moms-to-be when they take that breath, hold it, push and immediately break all the blood vessels in their faces. If you've heard of "face-pushing," or "pushing with your face," that's what we're talking about, and it's exhaustingly unproductive.

What seems to work better is to take the breath and, instead of holding it in your cheeks and face, sort of swallow it and hold the air in your lungs. Then, use the pressure of the air in your lungs as a brace against your lower abdominal and rectal muscles so you can bear down and push baby out of the birth canal. With this kind of pushing, even if you have an epidural, you can inch baby out without making your head explode.

The big moment is getting the head out because, of course, the head is the largest part of baby's anatomy. The crowning of baby's head creates a great deal of pressure and usually makes women feel the urge to bear down and push. In fact, when women are having their second, third, fourth, etc., birth, frequently the baby will be crowning–that is, the head will be right at the opening to the vagina–so you can reach down and feel his/her scalp before you even start to push.

When you have pushed your baby's head down so the opening of the vagina is stretched to its maximum, you will be experiencing what is known as "The Ring of Fire." If you have a drug-free birth, you may have a vivid story about why this is a good description. If you have an epidural, you will feel the greatest amount of pressure at this point while pushing the head out.* (*Please note, this description pertains to a regular head-down delivery. A breech presentation would have a different process and may result in a C-section).

Once the head comes out your OB will tell you to stop pushing for a minute so s/he can gently turn the baby's shoulders to an easier delivery position. Then one more push and baby will likely be out! Yay!!! Then, just after they get baby's shoulders out and remove baby from your body, you will know how the cows giving birth on Animal Planet feel. You know, the "MoooOOOO" and the "ka-THUMP" as they pull the calf out and the heifer just lies there all saggy and spent like a deflated hot air balloon? Yes. Only less fetching.

C-Sections

"I was shocked that you could be totally aware of what was going on and feel the tugging and pulling, but not experience any actual pain. That's seriously effed up." —Tracey B.

An emergency C-section is certainly something for which new moms wish they were better prepared. One third-time mom said:

"I hadn't even considered the possibility that I'd need a C-section, and felt thoroughly blindsided by the whole thing. However, it made me glad I had opted for the epidural because I don't know if they would have given me general anesthetic if I hadn't already had something in place. Baby T was out within 30 minutes of the doc calling a section... and I think mine was a pretty leisurely emergency C-section.

"I'll say one thing, though... I was shocked that you could be totally aware of what was going on and feel the tugging and pulling, but not experience any actual pain. That's seriously effed up." –Tracey B.

Seeing/Holding Baby for the First Time

Many moms confess feeling uncomfortable, worried and even frightened when they don't feel that instant, deep connection with their babies, but it's far more common than people acknowledge. Some relationships just take time... especially if one person is constantly screaming.

Frequently, new moms confess feelings of disconnection or detachment right after birth as they realize that as close as they felt to their babies during their pregnancies, these little people now seem like strangers. They are different than the fantasy babies many, many moms dreamed of from the first moment they saw two pink lines on a stick. Often new moms have a jumble of unexpected feelings—joy, distance, confusion, alienation, happiness, shock, disbelief—when they first hold their babies, but are afraid to show their true feelings to their partners.

This mixed bag of feelings can be stressful to new moms, especially if they've been told repeatedly that "you fall in love the moment you lay eyes on your baby," "it's a love unlike anything you've ever known," "you never knew you could love someone so much," "it's love at first sight," etc. Some moms confess feeling uncomfortable, worried or even frightened when they didn't experience the instant connection with their babies they had expected, but it's far more common than people acknowledge. Relationships can take time, especially when one person is constantly screaming.

One mother of three shared:

"When I had my first daughter, she was exactly what I expected—little, brown, beautiful. Bonding with her was effortless and immediate. The next time around could not have been more different. My second daughter started crying the moment she took her first breath, and DID NOT STOP CRYING FOR SIX WEEKS. I thought we'd made the biggest mistake of our lives having another baby, and it was the worst time in our marriage, too.

"Finally, whatever was wrong just went away and things got better. She was actually quiet for more than five seconds, and even started smiling. Once we came out of our catatonic state we were able to smile back, but it was really, really bad for a while there. We never figured out what was wrong—everyone just called it colic. It wasn't reflux or allergies or anything, but it certainly was nerve shredding, and it totally changed my expectations about bonding when I was pregnant with my third. I figured bonding and the newborn period would be whatever it was and we'd get through it somehow. I truly expected nothing, so anything positive was gravy."—Alicia F.

There are some people we click with right away and feel that instant connection. Other people can take more time to know, but the resulting bond is so true, real and deep, we can't imagine living without them. Feeling bonded to baby immediately probably makes the initial adjustment to parenthood easier, but the wonderment and humility of admitting that you are meeting your baby for the first time, and being ready to get to know him as a person, not just projecting a persona upon him, is a great beginning to a close, honest relationship.

Whatever your experience (or your husband/partner's experience) with initial bonding and attachment, most new moms recommend keeping realistic (a.k.a. "low") expectations. That way even if baby is screaming, wetting and covered with goo, you can still look back at those first moments and know that while it may not have been pretty, it was real. And real is healthy. Or, once again, you could go with a combination of denial and amnesia. Your choice.

Getting the Placenta Out

After baby comes out, your doctor will deliver your placenta, also known as the "afterbirth." Basically, the OB and the nurse (usually) semi-vigorously rub and massage your belly, working the placenta down the birth canal until you deliver it, too. You may be asked to push a couple times to finish the job. I've only experienced the afterbirth with the aid of a lingering epidural, and I felt pressure from the vigorous massaging, but it wasn't really painful.

Then the nurse will weigh your placenta. If you made plans to preserve your placenta, or if you recently decided you wanted to preserve your placenta, let the nurse and/or OB know right away.

Post-Birth Shock

Shaking, shivering, sweating, sweltering, starving, euphoria, racing thoughts and/or freezing to death can all be part of post-birth shock.

Many new moms are "shocked by the shock" and wish someone had told them that "getting baby out" wasn't the last major thing their bodies would experience on delivery day. Shaking, shivering, sweating, sweltering, starving, euphoria, racing thoughts and/or freezing to death can all be part of post-birth shock.

Some new moms were rather irked that their providers never mentioned post-birth shock. They reported feeling confused and unsettled by these post-birth sensations, and when the shock wasn't acknowledged, they only felt more confused about whether all the hot/cold/shaking/etc. was normal and when it would end.

Nurses will be at the ready with heated blankets to pile on you as soon as the shaking and shivering begin, but many new moms have trouble getting warm and may find this transition disconcerting. One mom said of her first birth experience:

"I was so relieved to be done with the delivery. My son was on my chest and the nurse picked him up to give him his first bath when suddenly I started to shake and shiver uncontrollably. My teeth were chattering—I even found it difficult to see. Not exactly blurred vision, but just totally disoriented for a few minutes. The nurse heard the bed rattling (from my shaking), and without even looking up from the baby's bath asked, 'Getting a little chilly?' 'Y-y-y-y-esssss,' I said through clenched teeth. Since her hands were wet she asked my husband to pile some heated blankets on me. I think he tucked in four or five before I started to feel better.

"While they were bathing my son I felt like I was on another planet. I could hear everyone talking to each other, but they sounded a million miles away and like they were speaking a foreign language. I didn't tell anyone because I didn't want to seem like a wimp. No one asked, 'Are you okay?' or said anything, so I just kept smiling so I wouldn't ruin the moment, but it would have been reassuring to hear someone say, 'You're experiencing post-birth shock. It's normal and should stop in about x minutes.'"—Rachel D.

Some women do not experience post-birth shock, or do not experience it with every birth. Dana was shocked that she *didn't* have post-birth shock after her fourth delivery when she always had before:

"I felt so relieved when I prepared to deliver my youngest that I finally knew what to expect. No more surprises! Then, for the first time in four births, I didn't have post-birth shock. What?! I had her at a different hospital, and their postnatal protocol allowed maximum skin-to-skin contact for mother and baby, so they didn't take her for a bath ten minutes after she was born like the others. Instead, they let the vernix (creamy white coating on baby) reabsorb into her skin, and didn't bathe her until hours later when I felt we were both ready.

I held her against my bare skin for our first eight hours together, and guess what? Not one shake, chatter or anything! I don't know if it was coincidence or not, but I always had had shock when they took the baby for the bath, and I wonder if holding her instead of physically separating us so soon after birth stopped me from having all those weird symptoms. Maybe Post-Birth Shock is a mother's hard-wired response to being apart from her baby too soon? Anyway, if there's a next time, no matter where I deliver, I'm going to hold the baby as long as I feel I need to. I believe it's best for both of us."–Dana M.

One more thing about post-birth symptoms: Usually within 24 hours of delivery women feel extremely hot and may begin to sweat profusely. This is the body's way of ridding itself of some of the excess fluid collected and stored during pregnancy, and for some women it feels a bit like being in your own mobile sauna.

Speaking for myself, after my first delivery the combination of the plastic hospital mattress, the heat of a nursing baby and South Florida-brand humidity was too much to bear politely. I finally couldn't take it anymore. When my husband called the next day on his way to visit us and asked if he could bring me anything (meaning food), I replied, "Either a fan or a window A/C unit." "But the hospital has central air," he said. I paused. "What's your point?"

First Breastfeeding Latch

This first breastfeeding experience does not accurately resemble what authentic breastfeeding may feel like from Postpartum Day 4 to about Day 30. You have been warned.

If you have had a vaginal birth, and are planning to breastfeed, your nurse/OB/midwife will likely encourage you to try to "breastfeed" as soon as possible after delivery. This first "breastfeeding" experience belongs in quotes because it does not accurately resemble what authentic breastfeeding may feel like from Postpartum Day 4 to about Day 30.

Quite a few new moms were shocked when they got home and found the "breastfeeding" that was going reasonably well in the hospital had taken on a whole different identity. We'll get to this more in Chapter 5, but just to give you a heads-up, here's the perspective of a first-time mom a couple days after "breastfeeding" in the hospital:

"I don't get it! Argh!!! The breasts I had two days ago are now rock-hard honeydews and my daughter's gums are like pliers. This was not in the books!!!" –Majni R.

What happens with you, your baby and your "girls" in the delivery room is more likely breastfeeding rehearsal or maybe just "latch practice." Initial latching is important for a bunch of reasons: Baby starts working those suckling muscles, mom's milk production starts to get the message, the colostrum (the nutrient-rich pre-milk) becomes stimulated to flow, and of course, the bonding of mother and baby is enhanced and supported by breastfeeding. Good stuff.

Yet, these are the very early pieces of the breastfeeding puzzle. Getting a good latch in the hospital is huge, and it is also only the beginning. Instead of believing that 48 hours of "breastfeeding in the hospital" encapsulates the entire breastfeeding experience, some moms found it helpful to understand a new mother's stages of breastfeeding. Below is *The Stages of Breastfeeding Adjustment* according to my observations–both personal and professional. Please know this is just one perspective:

Days 1-4: A little strange, feels like nothing's happening, hurts some.
Days 4-21: Milk comes in, engorgement ensues, latching on becomes moderately to extremely painful, good latch vital.
Days 21-30: Milk production is more under control, any continued problems are addressed with professional help, pain begins to ease, though still may require certain positions with certain props for comfort.
Days 30-beyond: Latching becomes essentially painless, good breastfeeding habits are established, mom continues to reach out for support.

Some moms found it helpful to approach early breastfeeding one session at a time for the first few months to avoid feeling overwhelmed.

If you know or are thinking that you may have a C-section, and breastfeeding is heavy on your mind, a good question to ask your provider could be this: "If I have a C-section (planned or unplanned), when would I likely be able to breastfeed?"

Immediate attempts at breastfeeding may not be possible with certain C-section situations. If you know or think you may have a C-section, at one of your many third trimester check-ups you could ask, "If I have a C-section (planned or unplanned), when would I *likely* (understanding birth guarantees aren't really realistic) be able to breastfeed?"

Some moms who gave birth by C-section were upset that they were not allowed to attempt breastfeeding right after their C-sections. Further, some felt the delay may have negatively affected bonding with their new babies. These observations are personal, of course, and not predictive of any other woman's experience.

One more thing on early breastfeeding: Most women who produce milk often see nothing coming from their breasts for the first 3 to 4 days, and may worry that they are not producing anything for their babies. If you are concerned, talk with your lactation consultant as soon as possible to determine if there is a problem and set your mind at ease.

Post-Birth Hunger

If it looks like you'll be delivering in the middle of the night, you may want to send your husband/partner/support person to the cafeteria during your labor to get you a meal for after delivery. And by a meal, I mean four courses. Minimum.

The feelings and sensations a woman experiences after delivery were touched on earlier in *Post-Birth Shock,* but one that deserves its own subsection is hunger. After delivery, women usually feel very, *very* hungry. This is one of those times when food tastes so good.

Be aware, however, if your baby is born between about 8 p.m. and 7 a.m. when most hospital cafeterias are closed, your menu choices could be limited to the vending machines. It's probably the last thing you'll be thinking of, but during your labor and while the cafeteria's open, you may want to send your husband/partner/support person to get you a meal for after delivery. And by a meal, I mean four courses. Minimum. I'm actually not kidding.

Episiotomies, Tearing & Stitches

Sometimes an episiotomy or a serious tear is unavoidable, and women are unpleasantly surprised by how these wounds and the resulting pain complicate their postpartum recoveries and "new baby" experiences in general. If you have to have an episiotomy, it's probably not what you'd hoped for, but you don't need to exhaust yourself by being upset about it. In a week or so, you will be fine. Maybe even sooner.

A common side-effect of narcotics is constipation. Many repeat moms say taking narcotics post-birth led to horrible constipation, so the next time they opted for Advil/Ibuprofen instead.

New moms with this inconvenient complication say what helped their psychological recovery most was good communication and reassurances that "in x days" they'd feel better, as well as having a good wound-care plan to guide them.

As far as wound care goes, some moms recovering from tears and episiotomies didn't know they could ask for steroid foam, witch-hazel (Tucks) pads and diaper ice packs in the hospital to ease their pain, and were pretty ticked when no one at their hospital offered. One second-time mom made her own diaper ice packs at home by soaking a maxi in water, putting it in a plastic bag, laying it curved in a pie tin and placing it in the freezer. It was a little more comfortable than a lump of ice jammed in her underpants.

If you have a 3rd or 4th degree tear or episiotomy, your postpartum nurse will likely offer you some kind of narcotic (Tylenol with Codeine or "T3," for example) for your pain. Let me say this, only you know how much pain you are in, and only you know what you need to feel remotely human. However, a common side-effect of narcotics is constipation, and if you have trauma to the "vaginanal" area, as one new mom called it, during birth, you probably don't want to have to strain when you use the bathroom and risk tearing your stitches or worse.

Instead of relying on narcotic painkillers, consider sticking with Advil/Ibuprofen, if you can stand it. The postpartum nurse may not mention that narcotics can cause constipation, but they can and the effects can be debilitating. Advil, Tucks and a diaper ice pack can be the best (least complicated) methods of delivery-wound care.

A Very Long Wheelchair Ride

If the ride is making your head swim, let the nurse know.
Many new moms feel uncomfortable asking for anything at this
point, but if it's bothering you, you have every right to speak up.
Maybe your partner can push instead. It doesn't hurt to ask.

I don't know exactly what happened, but the wheelchair ride from L&D to Postpartum Recovery after my first delivery felt like the terrifying nightmare Tim Robbins has in the '90s psychological thriller *Jacob's Ladder*. It just seemed to go on and on forever, with horrific images flying past at nauseatingly breakneck speed.

Maybe it was because the sun was going down and the shadows were strange. Maybe it was because the drugs were wearing off. Maybe it was because I was in an enormous county hospital with restricted sections and broken elevators and we had to cross a sky bridge to get to another wing and yadda, yadda, yadda. It took more than 20 minutes just to get to the floor below, but the whole journey was more than my battered body and soul could take at that moment. By the time I got to Postpartum Recovery, I was quaking and chattering. It was all I could do to crawl into bed, still feeling the motion in my stomach.

If they pile you into a wheelchair to move you from L&D to Postpartum Recovery, and you're sore from pushing, tearing and/or stitches, or groggy, nauseated or shaking and shivering from post-birth shock, feel free to ask the nurse to please, "Slow down." They are likely trying to get you to a bed, partly so you can rest and partly so they can pass off your care, so speed is the name of the game. Yet, if the ride is making your head swim, let the nurse know. Many new moms feel uncomfortable asking for anything at this point, but if it's bothering you, *you have every right to speak up.* Maybe your partner can push instead. It doesn't hurt to ask.

Some hospital maternity centers now have "LDR Rooms"— Labor, Delivery & Recovery, so you don't have to go on a midnight ride with your arse on fire. If you deliver in an LDR Room, the farthest you'll have to trek is the bathroom, which is another brand of terror, but at least it doesn't occur at 35 miles per hour.

CHAPTER 4

INITIAL RECOVERY

That Just Happened

So... *congratulations!!!* You've just given birth! Wow, can you believe it? One moment the baby is inside, and the next she's out breathing on her own and in your arms. Finally, after so many months, you get to see each other, touch each other and begin to get to know each other as you actually are. You've been dreaming of this mystery person for months, and I think, in her own way, she's being dreaming of you, too.

Whether it's your first, second or fifth delivery, giving birth is pretty astonishing, and now that it's over you can... um... well... take a chair because you have nine months of baby-baking to unwind. It took approximately 40 weeks to get to this miracle and it's going to take 40 (or more) to come down from it and find a new you.

Your doctor may tell you you can resume all normal activities six weeks after delivery (mostly meaning exercise, lifting things and sex). However, over the last couple decades this boilerplate advice has mushroomed into a myth about modern motherhood that goes a little something like this... (Ahem), "A new mom can resume all 'normal activity' within six weeks, presumably including (but not limited to) returning to work, exercise, friendships, cute clothes, party-throwing, coherent conversation, being pleasant and, of course, not just *having* sex but *enjoying it*." Ha! My oldest is eight, and I'm still waiting to resume my "normal activities." Any day now.

Maybe this myth been packaged differently for you, but you've likely heard or read something similar to the above. It's pervasive, persistent, and just plain stupid. I mean, really... name any other life-altering adjustment after which a person is expected to just resume "normal activities." Does anyone ever say to a 20-year-old woman, "Phew! Well, now that adolescence is over, you can get back to playing with your Barbie dolls. After all, the whole 'transition to adulthood' thing was just a phase, right?"

You can't "go back" to anything. Like trying to return to a childhood hideout after years of absence, when we try to stuff ourselves back into molds we've outgrown, we often find that, though we recognize everything, it doesn't fit or feel the same. You may or may not have spent time before birth–or before pregnancy–thinking about the pre-baby you–acknowledging the impending change, processing and letting go, but you're not alone. How can any of us ever truly understand or prepare for the bright line of Life Before Baby and Life After Baby?

You need to know your partner likely won't experience the "Before Baby/After Baby" life change the same way you do. Your husband's/partner's life does change, certainly, but not like yours. His life changes because *you* change, but it's much different for him. Is it fair? Well, we know life's not fair, but that's not really what it's about, is it? It's about discovering the best that each of us can be. If we only strive to be "even" with everyone else, we really shortchange ourselves.

So, now here you are, and it's amazing. You've given birth to a new life for a baby, a family and a new life for you, too. You are a mother now, and, as is true with every major life transition, you are taking in *and* letting go. It's okay to feel happy and sad about those changes, even at the same time. No new life stage is all ecstatic exuberance. No matter what you see on Facebook.

Bleeding & Cheesecloth Underpants

When it comes to birth and postpartum recovery modesty goes right out the window. The only goal is survival. No matter how "natural" a process giving birth is, it is still a trauma in certain ways, and while you're shuffling around in cheesecloth underpants with everyone and their medical student checking the status of your junk for a few days, just know "This too shall pass."

After you give birth, you are going to bleed a lot, so much so that you will likely need super-human maxi pads that do not fit in regular underwear. It seems that everyone but postpartum patients know this unpleasant inevitability. After you deliver and before you can protest, your nurse will unceremoniously pass you a pair of cheesecloth underpants into which you are supposed to jam the mattress pad, I mean the maxi pad, the witch-hazel wipes and (God-willing) your diaper ice pack. And then sit down. And attempt to breastfeed. Oh, and "relax." Riiiight.

This awkward moment isn't meant to humiliate, yet I know many, *many* women who would have appreciated a feeling of "Ah, yes, the cheesecloth underpants... I've been expecting you," as they flop into a pair with every Kimberly-Clark product in the Western World stuck to their crotches. Instead, there we are, disposable underwear in hand, hunching by the hospital bed, trying to simply engage our atrophied and anesthetized leg muscles enough to get our big toes into these babies.

Why do we not mention basic postpartum recovery protocol to women at their final OB appointments? Does it seem unimportant? Do we not want to scare them? As one mom said:

"I would really have liked a heads-up on the granny-panties and insane maxi pads. I sent my mom to Target from the hospital to buy XL underwear so I could shuffle around the hospital without dropping trou every few feet. I would much rather someone had told me to just bring huge underwear to the hospital. It's not like it was a surprise to my doctor or nurse! For God's sake, when you're taking my blood pressure for the five millionth time (not saying that's not important, but stay with me), please just slip that info in there so I won't be caught, literally, with my pants down!" –Kelley H.

Soreness & Diaper Ice Packs

You can keep asking for diaper ice packs as often as you want—no need to wait for the nurse to offer one. Only you know what you need.

If you have a vaginal delivery, you are going to have a sore bottom, though how sore depends on multiple factors. Some new moms have remarked that after the first 12 hours post-birth, the postpartum nurses stopped offering diaper ice packs. Half believing this was protocol and half not wanting to be a bother, these moms didn't ask for more diaper ice packs when they still really needed them. Truth time: *You can keep asking for diaper ice packs as often as you want—no need to wait for the nurse to offer.*

Also, ibuprofen, Ben Gay/Icy Hot-type topical ointments (check with your OB first, to be safe) and hot showers can help relieve muscle soreness. You probably won't be cleared for baths for a while, but hot water from a shower can provide some relief (and help make peeing and other things easier–it's all drains) in the beginning. Furthermore, as one mom said, *"The shower is a great place to cry,"* so you're really multi-tasking. Bravo.

If you're so sore you can't even sit, you can try nursing baby lying down in bed. One postpartum nurse gave me so much grief about doing this with my first, it nearly brought me to tears. She told me I was going to "give that baby an ear infection." Fortunately, my husband, who was an ENT (Ear, Nose & Throat) resident physician at the time, came in at the tail end of my scolding and heard her prophecy of doom. "Don't worry," he whispered to me. "She's not coming home with us."

Recovery from C-Sections

A C-section recovery comes with some unique issues. A mom of three shared this about her C-section recovery following her third birth:

"The recovery period nearly drove me insane. Thankfully, my OB cleared me to drive once I was off the narcotic, so I weaned myself off within a week and was driving the big kiddos to and from school by Day 10 postpartum. However, you're not allowed to lift anything heavier than the baby for six weeks (some sources say 4-6 weeks, so I was doing a little bit of stuff around 4/5 weeks). That includes not lifting a gallon of milk (which weighs about 10 lbs.) no vacuuming and no carrying laundry baskets. The last two nearly did me in. With a family of five and a dog, vacuuming and laundry are a near-daily occurrence. Not being able to do those things was out of control.

"Oh, even if you deliver by C-section, still take the Colace. My hemorrhoids were on fire following delivery, probably due to the fact that I still pushed for quite a while before the section was called. And, the surgery itself slows down your bowel function, so you'll want things to stay nice and soft as function returns."

"I have to admit the C-section was NOT as painful as a 4th degree vaginal tear, and I felt much better much sooner than I expected (which just added to my not-allowed-to-clean frustration)."–Tracey B.

Pain Medication

It's tempting to take narcotic painkillers like Tylenol with Codeine (T3) or Percocet when the epidural wears off and the pain really hits, but narcotics will slow digestion and constipate you even more than the epidural already has. Considering how sore your bottom may be, as well as any perineal wounds you're dealing with, you may want to steer clear of *anything* that could further constipate you. Many new moms regretted loading up on narcotics during their hospital stays because they wound up paying the piper once they got home.

Following my first birth, my postpartum night nurse told me that Colace (stool softener) or Milk of Magnesia would "fix everything," and insisted I just "take the narcotics" for the pain from my fourth-degree episiotomy. The net result? Ten long, nauseating, yellow days without a bowel movement.

It still confounds me that in all four of my postpartum hospital stays only *one* postpartum nurse ever came clean that: 1. Narcotics constipate, and 2. It may be better for a woman to stick to Ibuprofen, if she can, or alternate narcotics and ibuprofen. Women are often raised to be agreeable and follow directions, so if a caregiver tells us to do something, we usually do it with few or no questions—especially if we're in pain. Thus, when I was presented with T3 after my first birth I never thought to ask, "What are the side effects? Can I take something else?" I just figured, "They do this all time. They're the professionals. Just do as you're told."

It's not easy to know what to do or take when you're feeling awful. Bottom line, *being in agony with pain does not help anyone*—you need to do what's best for you. My only point is that many new moms say they wish they'd known they could try a lower dose of narcotics, or only use ibuprofen after delivery, so they didn't end up with uncomfortable side effects later.

Walking

I know that long walk was too much of a strain for me less than 24 hours after birth. I can't believe no one stopped me. Rookie mistake.

Okay, now you're thinking, "Walking? *Walking??* What kind of an idiot does this person think I am? Yeah, I get it; it's going to be tough to walk right after birth. Thanks for the newsflash. Sheesh, moron." Yes, I know you know that—and if you didn't, you would have figured it out pretty fast—but this isn't about just "walking." This is about pacing yourself as you start walking after birth. Short, easy walks, not long, adventurous sojourns. One mom's experience with walking after birth really took her by surprise:

"My son's head was so big—the 95th percentile compared to his height and weight, which was in the 50th—that the team wanted to make sure he didn't have hydrocephalus, (a.k.a. "water on the brain"). They ordered an MRI for him the day after he was born. The imaging center where the MRI would be performed was two wings and one tower away (about a 20-minute walk) through the sprawling urban hospital where I delivered.

"Because he was my 1-day-old baby, I insisted on going with him to the MRI. Further, because I was still so sore from pushing and my episiotomy, I could not sit down in a wheelchair, so I walked the whole 20-minute walk, pushing his isolette the whole way, like a walker, for balance.

"By the time we got there I didn't feel very well, and just before it was time to return to my room (he was fine—just a large head), I started to feel dizzy from the pain and fatigue of such a long walk, and nearly passed out. My husband had to find a gurney to take me back to my room so I could lie down. I know that long walk was too much of a strain for me to attempt less than 24 hours after birth. I can't believe no one stopped me."—Gracie W.

More Diaper Ice Packs

This is probably a good time for another one. I'll wait.

Postpartum Nurses

If you feel stressed or pushed around, don't be afraid to have someone advocate for you. This is about your recovery, not someone else's agenda.

I want to say right up front that I have had the pleasure to know and be cared for by some *wonderful* postpartum nurses. However, I have also personally observed and heard from many, many other new moms that *some* (again, by no means *all*) postpartum nurses, though they work very hard to meet the needs of so many new moms and babies, sometimes bring vibes of impatience and irritation to the postpartum recovery room that leave new moms feeling stressed out and incompetent rather than relaxed and supported.

This can be a shock after having a good rapport with the L&D nurse, and several new mothers have said they wish someone had warned them to be on guard and advocate for themselves while in Postpartum Recovery. If your postpartum nurses start (unintentionally) stressing you out with schedules, questions and demands, not to mention 5 a.m. shift changes (which is definitely an ideal time for chit chat), don't be afraid to speak up and/or have someone advocate for you, especially if you feel the nurses are irritated with you for asking questions, breastfeeding on your side(!) or refusing to do a Sitz bath (more on that shortly). This is about your recovery, not someone else's agenda.

Lactation Consultants

If you do not click with your lactation consultant and/or feel pressured, judged, intimidated, misunderstood or that she is drifting into "boob nazi" territory and you're starting to break out in hives at the sound of her voice, you can "break-up" with her and find a more rewarding "lactational relationship." You are not responsible for anyone else's self-esteem at this point. Your job is to take care of you and your baby. Period.

You can expect a visit from the lactation consultant on duty within the first two to eight hours after giving birth. The postpartum nurses usually have the experience and knowledge to help you with early feeding issues, but working with a specialist who has more one-on-one time to spend with you and your baby can be invaluable. Many lactation consultants are absolutely phenomenal—knowledgeable, encouraging, friendly and down-to-earth. Most lactation consultants I have known really love what they do and are only too glad to help you and your baby get off to a great start with breastfeeding.

Some new moms, however, are surprised by the (seeming) ever-presence of the lactation consultant, and may find her ongoing input to be an invasion of privacy and personal space. I can understand this point of view. I mean, they look at your boobs, handle your boobs, examine your boobs, etc. I started to feel like I was at the boob mechanic—"So ma'am, how've the old girls been runnin' lately? Do they sputter in the mornin'? Any leaks?" All this while they very hurriedly and matter-of-factly rifle around "under the hood," so to speak.

Most often, though, it's not a big deal. Over the last 10 years I've worked with eight different lac consultants, and the experiences have been pretty simple and consistent. She'll chit chat for a moment and then quickly get to, "Has s/he latched on yet? Yes? Oh good, and for how long? Yes? And the other side, how did that go? Good, good." Then she'll ask if you have any questions, and if you, by chance, happen to be nursing your baby when she is there, she'll check on baby's latching and, nine times out of 10, give in to her well-intentioned urge to shove some pillows under your elbows.

One second-time mom recently shared this about her experience with lactation consultants:

"At many or, perhaps, most, community hospitals, you can ask for the lactation consultant to come and see you anytime. She may be busy and you'll have to wait for a bit, and the nurses can help you with immediate feeding issues, but you can always ask for another visit from the lactation consultant as long as you are in the hospital. After you leave the hospital you can call the lactation consultant and leave a message and she'll return your call within 24 hours, or schedule a time to meet with her if you have any questions at all. Some community hospitals even offer a free postpartum home-visit from a lactation consultant, and most women I know who've utilized the service say it is a life-saver, not just for feeding issues, but postpartum in general."–Kelley H.

Not everyone knows about these home visits, or unlimited access to lac consultants, and each hospital does things a little differently, so be sure to find out exactly what the breadth of lactation services are, and use them. Overall, lac consultants *love* helping new moms breastfeed, strive to be available and are quick to respond when moms reach out.

If you do not click with yours and feel pressured, judged, intimidated or misunderstood, *break-up with her and find someone else.* Most mid-sized to large hospitals have at least two lactation consultants in rotation at any time, and you are free to wait for/or specifically ask for the other one. And if you like your nurse, but you don't click with either one of the lactation consultants, you can ask your nurse breastfeeding questions and/or investigate your local La Leche League and other breastfeeding resources in your community.

You may want more from the lactation consultant, you may want less, and you'll figure it out, but many moms agree the interaction with the lactation consultant is another surprising example of how, as a mother, your body is no longer your own. Your breasts are no longer sexual. (Well, they still are to some people, but that's another topic.) They are as functional as a soda fountain. They make milk, and for the foreseeable future, that's their primary purpose, despite what your bewildered husband/partner attempts to grope to the contrary.

Safety & Security Policies

If you do the maternity wing/hospital tour, your guide can be a good person to ask about Safety & Security in Postpartum Recovery. This is not likely to be your OB's area of expertise.

Any hospital worth its salt is going to have safety policies in place and I don't mean stuff like, "Lift with your legs, not with your back." I mean safety policies about who can take your baby out of your room, when they can take baby and where baby goes. Many new moms are surprised that this can be a complicated issue, and it can cause extra and unnecessary stress if it's sort of piled on you when you're already oscillating between post-birth euphoria and new-parent anxiety.

You may ask about your chosen hospital's Safety & Security Policies at any time if that is important to you, as well as the hospital's record for maternal/infant safety and security. If you do the maternity wing/hospital tour, your guide may be a good person to ask about Safety & Security in Postpartum Recovery. This is not likely to be your OB's area of expertise.

If you do not ask ahead of time (I certainly didn't–it never even crossed my mind), know that you are free to ask anytime. The standard protocol at most institutions seems to be that *anyone* who is authorized to take your baby out of your room/away from your supervision during your hospital stay _must_ have a certain color name badge and/or other official hospital-issued photo identification.

Some hospitals are so small and intimate, security isn't really an issue, but for moms who give birth at urban, public and teaching hospitals which tend to be large, bureaucratic institutions, understanding Postpartum Recovery Safety & Security Policies may be very important to their overall comfort. One mom said this about her postpartum experience at a public hospital in a major U.S. city:

"My husband had been employed by the hospital as a resident for more than two years, so the whole thing seemed comfortably familiar. I felt good about the care and the competence of the attending physicians and residents, yet I never, ever considered how different it would feel to be a patient there. It was a public county hospital. It was enormous, included seven different freestanding hospitals on the campus and was dedicated to serving the underserved, so there were many safety and security problems I simply never imagined... until I was stuck there, literally unable to flee.

"A few weeks before I delivered our oldest child, there had been a baby-snatching at the hospital. A newborn was kidnapped right out of the Neonate Nursery. It was horrifying. Because of that disaster, the administrators had put in place a bunch of new, super-strict Safety & Security Policies. There were two armed policemen at the double doors to the Postpartum/Neonate wing, and you had to show photo ID and sign in to visit any postpartum patient.

"Upon arriving at the Postpartum floor, the nurses gave us strict written and verbal instructions not to let anyone watch, hold, take or touch our babies, unless that person had a hospital-issued PINK Photo Name Badge with corresponding Photo ID to match. We were not to leave the baby in our rooms even if we went to the bathroom or to take a shower. We were to call a nurse to take the baby to the Nursery until we were back in bed.

"I was glad on one hand that the hospital was taking the kidnapping so seriously, and I guess I felt safer in a way, but mostly I felt terrified! You can guess how long I tried to wait between trips to the bathroom. With all that hullabaloo, I wasn't completely certain I even trusted the <u>nurse</u> to take my son to the Nursery. I mean, what if she took her eyes off him for a moment? I just wanted to get out of there.

"The second morning we were there someone came in my room and asked to take my baby for his hearing test, but she wasn't wearing a PINK Name Badge. When I asked her about it she sheepishly replied, 'I was afraid you'd ask me that... I left it in my office. Do you want me to go get?' 'Yes,' I answered, but I was kind of ticked. Why would she even ask to take him without her name badge when she knew that was the hospital's new policy? Didn't she know what kind of position that put an exhausted, increasingly anxious new mother in?

"All the other hospitals I've delivered in, and there have been several, have not been at all like what I experienced in the inner-city. I'm so sorry that any new mothers have to go through that kind of militant security on top of everything else." –Gracie W.

Hospital Safety & Security may not be an issue for you, and I wish it weren't for anyone, but for Gracie W., myself and others, the safety aspect became another worry (and a frightening one) following an exhausting delivery. I wish I'd known what I was getting my baby and myself into before I delivered at the public county hospital. I would have asked a friend or family member to stay with me around the clock.

As Gracie further said:

"I was afraid to nod off even for a moment for fear I'd wake up and my baby would be missing. It was just more worry than I could take." –Gracie W.

The Postpartum Parade

Knwalk: (Verb) Def. To knock mid-stride while walking into a Postpartum Recovery room without awaiting a response.

I had no idea how many people can stream in and out of one hospital room over two days, and many other new moms I've met agree the two recovery days in the hospital can feel a lot like going to a cocktail party in your pajamas. Honestly, from four in the morning to past midnight the following day, there was someone "knwalking" (my term for the entry/greeting on the Postpartum Floor,) at least every hour, if not more.

I don't mean to complain. The nurses and other staff have assignments and protocols to follow, and I'm truly grateful for their diligent care. That said, for those who need peace and quiet to recharge after something as life-altering as, you know, *giving birth*, the Postpartum Parade may feel like a lot of interaction, enthusiasm and interruptions.

Hopefully, you will not feel the need to spend extra energy on being kind or, God-forbid, witty with anyone. Yet, if you are the type of person that likes to be thoughtful and nice and ask other people how their day is going, just be warned that you will meet *a lot* of new friends in those 48 hours, and it may start to feel slightly (or extremely) draining.

More visits from more people—clinical, lay and social—go on into the night, and all the while your boobs spend more time outside your pj top than in, but who could blame them? They've never seen a show like this!

If you give birth in the night, the first person you will likely see before the sun rises is the postpartum nurse, followed by the pediatrician around 7 a.m. Then the rounding OB/Gyn physician may drop by, followed by the lactation consultant, then, perhaps, someone from hospital human resources or quality control. Hopefully, at some point someone brought you a meal or two, and most likely at least one of the housekeeping staff has come through to empty the wastebaskets along with maintenance to change a light bulb. Probably when one or both of your "girls" are roaming free.

Now your nurse has come again–she needed to tie up loose ends before her shift change. Then, the new nurse comes in to say hello and check on you. Next, maybe another visit from the lactation consultant, then the audiologist for baby's hearing screening, followed by the newborn photographer peddling her wares, and, of course, excited family and friends drifting in (or maybe more like "plunking down") throughout the day. Fingers crossed that someone has, once again, brought you more food. Visits from every corner–clinical, lay and social–go on into the night, and all the while your boobs have a front row seat, spending more time outside your nursing top than in.

Meanwhile, you try to maintain a shred of dignity while you shuffle to the bathroom, bravely facing nature's call, then shuffle back to bed, trying not to knock into the isolette where baby–possibly the only person *not* getting on your nerves at this point–is sleeping through the whole circus. All of this is gracefully accomplished with both a diaper full of ice and maxi-pad fit for Trampoline World stuffed into your very own figure-flattering cheesecloth underpants.

Somewhere in the midst of this familiar scene, someone will ask you, "Hey, are you okay? Do you want us to go so you can get some sleep?" And just as you force a weak smile to take him/her up on the offer, you hear a knwalk and swiftly moving squeaks on the linoleum... "Hey, how are we doing? I just need a minute..."

Trying to Sleep at the Hospital

It may not be possible to actually "rest" in the hospital, despite your best efforts. It's not just you.

Why is this section entitled "Trying to Sleep at the Hospital" and not "*Sleeping* at the Hospital"? Please see *The Postpartum Parade* section.

Seriously, many new moms find that actually *sleeping* at the hospital is very difficult, and instead may end up nodding off while sitting in bed trying to nurse their babies. Some moms say packing their own pillows helped, and one mom advocated bringing a sleep mask since it's never really "dark" in a hospital room with the hallway light drifting in and monitors glowing, to say nothing of roommates, partners and assorted TVs and tablets.

It may not be possible to actually "rest" in the hospital, which can further deepen your post-birth exhaustion. No quick fix for this—just know your mental state is intricately intertwined with your physical state, so if you start feeling awful in your head, it likely means you need more rest for your body, and you may need to leave the hospital to get it

One last thing on rest and exhaustion, if at any time you start having thoughts that worry or scare you, reach out for help immediately. Get a referral from your provider for a mental-health professional *who is experienced in perinatal/postpartum mental health complications*. You are likely experiencing "intrusive thoughts," a common and disturbing symptom of Postpartum Obsessive-Compulsive Disorder.

Postpartum OCD is an expression of Postpartum Distress and is frequently triggered by exhaustion/sleep deprivation. Women who experience this symptom often fear they are "going crazy," but remember this–if you're *afraid* you're going crazy, you're probably not *actually going* crazy. If the scary thoughts seemed to make sense to you and you were in the midst of making a *plan* to act on the scary thoughts, that would be different. That would be a sign of *Postpartum Psychosis, an extremely serious perinatal mental health complication that requires immediate medical attention.*

Please know this–*no matter how bad things may seem, it is never hopeless.* Postpartum mental-health issues are highly treatable if addressed. Do not conceal your true feelings and worries. If you are having thoughts that scare you, please reach out for help immediately. You can go to www.postpartum.net and find local help from peer support providers and get information about local professionals who understand Postpartum Distress complications. You are not alone, no matter how you feel. There is help. *You are not alone*.

The Sitz Bath

If you are too worn out to argue with a nurse who is all over you like a cheap suit about the Sitz bath, enlist reinforcements. Husbands are pretty good at drawing the line, and new grandmas are awesome at it. You want to talk Mama Bear? Get Grandma on the scene.

What is a "Sitz Bath" you ask? It's a basin of warm water made to fit on the toilet seat so you can soak your poor, abused hindquarters. Most hospitals don't have bathtubs in the postpartum rooms so often a Sitz Bath is encouraged (or demanded!) in your first 24 hours post-birth.

Some women really like these, especially if they've had an episiotomy or tearing because a Sitz Bath can be soothing to the wound and relaxing for the sore muscles. However..., *you do not have to do a Sitz bath.* That is up to you, and I don't give a flying fig if it's on someone's checklist! (Clearly, this hits home for me). If you are so sore you can't sit down on the toilet, too tired to get up and go to the bathroom, or just want to be left the #@%# alone, that is A-Okay, and you should not have to take any flak about it.

If you are too worn out to argue with a nurse who is all over you like a cheap suit about the Sitz bath, enlist reinforcements. Partners/husbands can be very good at drawing the line, and new grandmas are *awesome* at it. You want to talk Mama Bear? Get the newly minted Grandma on the scene.

If no one else is around to fight this battle for you, here's a way out: Tell the nurse that you'll do the Sitz Bath after 7—either a.m. or p.m.—because that's usually the nursing shift change, and then tell the next nurse you did it after the last one left. Or, if you like this nurse better, tell her you *didn't* do it and you're not going to, so get over it, and you'll both have a good laugh.

Regardless, the whole thing is ridiculous. I wish I had known it's okay to think it's ridiculous, and just say, "No." The purpose of meds, ice packs, creams, checking wounds, lactation consultants and Sitz baths is to aid in *your* recovery, so if you aren't ready for something, need more information or just plain don't want to do it, let your team know and do what you need to do to feel well.

Hospital Food

I know you're thinking, "There she goes, beating the bathroom drum again." Well, you're not wrong.

Just another nod to the ongoing post-birth battle with constipation and regularity. Many hospitals have great food, and more than likely you will be *extremely* hungry after not eating for a day (or more) during labor and delivery. Further, if you suffered indigestion, acid reflux, nausea and more during pregnancy, this may be your first chance in a long time to eat, enjoy and even retain a meal! Yay!

A word of caution before you pick up the phone for your well-deserved feast, hospital food is frequently prepared with processed ingredients—including white sugar, salt and partially hydrogenated oils (ironic, isn't it?), all of which may further constipate you. I know you're thinking, "There she goes, beating the bathroom drum again–enough already!" While I may be a broken record on this, it is only because I care. Ten days without a bowel movement was a very "unfun" problem to endure post-delivery, and the wretched experience has made me a believer in whole, high-fiber foods just before and after birth.

Another Word on Diaper Ice Packs

Did you get another one the last time we talked about this? I'm not trying to get all Sitz-bathy on you, and if you don't want one that is your prerogative, but if you didn't get one because you're feeling too exhausted to ask, or you're sick and tired of people coming in your room but honestly know it would make you feel better, I encourage you to take a minute and get one.

If you keep a steady stream of ice packs going so that area stays more or less numb, you won't have to deal with that unpleasant, nauseating, up and down feeling of "pain/relief/pain/relief." It's totally up to you, but much like Colace, you really can't have too many diaper ice packs. Go ahead and take a minute to think it over, and get another one, if you like. I'll wait.

Older Children & Visitors

I felt too guilty and embarrassed to tell my husband and parents that I wanted them to take the kids home so they could play and I could rest.

We talked a bit about visitors in the *Postpartum Parade* section a few pages back, and how having visitors can be exhausting and make it more difficult to sleep, nurse and begin to physically recover, but there's something a lot of moms don't know that they wish someone had told them—*you are allowed to tell people to leave.*

Whether they will listen is another kettle of fish, but you can even plot with your nurse to come in around a certain time and shoo everyone out, "Doctor's orders! Time for the patient to rest!" (Your doctor will be the most wonderful scapegoat through quite a bit of the recovery process and will issue all sorts of edicts about your health and recovery that s/he never even knows about and doesn't have to, if you catch my drift).

After a good friend had her third child, she revealed:

"I thought I would be dying to see my older children and show them their new little sister—we'd been waiting so long for her! But after about 10 minutes of holding, rocking and taking pictures, they were over it and so was I.

"They wanted to make the bed go up and down (which made my stomach turn), and watch cartoons (which also kind of made my stomach turn—I didn't want any extra noise on. Everything already seemed overly loud). Finally, my mother took them to the cafeteria and the nurses gave them paper airplanes, but they stayed for more than two hours, and I felt too guilty and embarrassed to tell my husband and parents to take the kids home so they could play and I could rest with the new baby.

"I needed space and time to heal a bit. If I'd had surgery unrelated to having a baby, no one would have dreamed of bringing two children to visit me at the hospital for two hours. However, because it was a new baby, and everyone's excited about the new baby, it becomes this special family moment where the children come and have the first meeting with their new brother or sister.

"It is an extraordinary moment. But past the "moment" it's just Mommy game-on as usual, and Mommy is most decidedly benched at the moment. Actually, Mommy has left the Building."–Erin S.

The key word there is "moment." Some new moms have dreamt of sharing this beautiful moment with those they love–especially their older children–for so long, they don't think to create an exit strategy. Friends, relatives and children may not pick up on your hints and cues because they can't imagine how you're feeling. It may be up to you to draw the line on the "moment" and ask your visitors to leave.

If you're uncomfortable with giving your loved ones the heave ho, you may want to consider planning the visit before they come, rather than leaving it open-ended. Some moms suggested telling your family and friends you "can't wait to see them *and* you're also really exhausted, so could they come for about 20 minutes (it'll end up being at least a half-hour), then go out to lunch/to the store with Daddy/Grandma, and if they have time, stop by for one more hug on the way home?"

Speaking for myself, I had no idea having my family at the hospital for more than 20 minutes would be so overwhelming to me, but I learned–give instructions for the Big Sib moment, prepare for the moment, and enjoy the moment, then say goodbye, lie down, and stare out the window with a vacant expression. Until the next knwalk, that is.

Peeing

The only way I can describe the sensation of the primary post-birth urination is to say that it felt like my bladder was trying to throw up.

The first attempt at peeing after delivery is often not pretty. I still could not tell you exactly what occurred the first time I peed after giving birth. The feeling had just come back in my legs after my epidural, and the nurse said I needed to "void" (a.k.a. "pee") before I could go to Postpartum Recovery. Looking back, I would have been wise to refuse to pee and just stay there in L&D where that hospital's nurses were far more pleasant. However, eager to please, I hobbled over to the bathroom and did as I was told.

The only way I can describe the sensation of the first post-birth urination is that it felt like my bladder was trying to throw up. Things kept stopping and starting in this bizarre and somewhat painful undulating rhythm I couldn't control. The closest comparison would be a severe UTI, which makes sense since your bladder is so severely compressed during birth that it becomes, in one OB's words, "Traumatized." Lovely.

The nurses asked if I "was able to void." I meekly replied, "Yes," and kept the rest of my questions and concerns to myself. I was still basking in the glow of having survived birth without splitting down the middle like a codfish, and wasn't interested in tarnishing my gleaming moment with unpleasant realities such as, "Yes, from now on, when you pee, it will feel like your bladder is trying to throw up."

That Which Often Accompanies Peeing

*If you are too sore to sit on the toilet, you can always have a
bowel movement in the shower. I'm not saying it's a happy
thought, but the alternative of nothing is definitely worse.*

Much has been said about this topic in many other places,
and I really am aiming only to share what other women wish they'd
known before giving birth, not gross you out, so I will keep this
discussion brief.

Surviving/enduring a bowel movement in the first six weeks
post-birth may require that you "go to your happy place," and the
first bathroom experience after delivery can be flat-out painful. If
you are too sore to sit on the toilet, please know many women end
up "going" in the shower. The warm water is relaxing and can help
"move things along." I know this is disgusting, but I promised truth,
not beauty, and at least you know I'm not holding out on you.

Unexpected Bonding Issues & Concerns

*Wanting to "run away" from something unexpected and/or
frightening can be a normal human reaction. The key to
working through it is to talk about it with someone you trust.*

As we said in Chapter 3, bonding is a process, and that process changes when the situation with your baby is not what you expected. Difficulty bonding is one of the hardest things a new parent can experience.

Many new mothers feel terribly guilty for having negative thoughts about their newborns–how they look, how they cry, how they respond to their parents, as well as more complex issues like unexpected health concerns and more. New parents under this kind of stress may experience escape fantasies and/or impulses to run away (also a common symptom of Postpartum Distress–see Chapter 5 "Postpartum Stress & Distress" for more).

When they are able to talk about their feelings, new parents are relieved to know that other loving moms and dads have felt similar mixed emotions and *things usually get better*. Of course, there are no quick fixes to some difficult situations. There may be an adjustment period while you, your partner, your pediatrician and other supportive adults in your life begin learning about your baby and what s/he needs to thrive.

Difficulty bonding and unexpected concerns can create a confusing mix of feelings for new parents, and that is normal. The key to dealing with those feelings is to *talk about them with someone you trust*. There are people in your life and beyond to support you at this challenging time so you can find a good way forward for yourself and your family.

New Dads

Some people–dads, yes, but moms, too–can't (and don't) live at a fever pitch of emotion for more than a couple hours, tops. It's just too draining on them.

Some new moms are surprised, disappointed or even downright ticked when their husbands, now new dads, spend as much time "screen-sucking" (a.k.a., messing around with their iWhatevers) as they do paying attention to their recovering wives and new babies.

This can be annoying, especially if you've seen other dads go absolutely bananas over their new babies, or heard stories about how "… wonderful and thoughtful so-and-so was after I delivered–he brought me food, flowers and jumped up every time the baby made a sound. He didn't want to put her down for a second!" Or worse still, are reading from your hospital bed some incredibly heartfelt confession of gratitude and wonderment from a brand new dad on Facebook as you watch your husband/partner play Candy Crush on his handheld for the five millionth time.

Again, it's all about expectations. Some people–dads, yes, but moms, too–can't sustain such intense emotions for more than a couple of hours, tops. It's too draining. It could be that your husband/partner is so overwhelmed with the enormity of birth and fatherhood that he needs some time to himself to recharge. Playing a mindless game, texting with a friend or watching sports on TV–having no idea the noise is driving you crazy–may be just what he needs to get his balance back after the emotions of the last few days.

Relationships are built moment by moment over days, weeks and years. New moms need not interpret new dads' lack of utter fascination with their babies (and, let's be honest, their wives) as disinterest. He just may need time and space to regroup.

One more thing, not everyone is a "baby person." Many moms envision certain reactions from their babies' dads that may or may not occur. This unfulfilled expectation can be disappointing and feel hurtful. In Group, we talk sometimes about noticing the good that *is* happening, rather than what is *not* happening, and appreciating the unique positives each parent brings to the family.

Circumcision

If you're planning to have the little guy circumcised, find out in the first day whether the Pedi or the OB will be doing it, and how long you will have to stay afterward. This communication breakdown held us up for seven extra hours with one of the crankiest nurses I've ever known when our oldest was born.

With our second son, we had the procedure done first thing in the morning of the second day to allow him time to recover and get cleared for discharge. A large improvement.

The NICU

Many new moms whose newborns spent time in the NICU wished they had known the protocol for supporting breastfeeding during a NICU stay.

Having your newborn in the *Neonatal Intensive Care Unit*, or NICU [NIK-you], can be frightening, frequently unexpected and extremely stressful for the new parents. Many new moms whose babies spent time in the NICU following delivery said they wished they had asked more questions about the NICU when they were pregnant.

To be specific, some new moms wish they'd asked whether their delivering hospitals had a NICU, what sort of health problems would require transfer to a larger NICU at a different hospital, whether their babies could breastfeed while in the NICU, if they should bring a pump and leave bottled breastmilk for the nurses to administer and whether they could hold their babies in the NICU.

One mom had this to say about her baby's NICU stay:

"I wish someone had told me what would happen with my baby's feeding in case we landed in the NICU! I never thought it would happen, but it did. Since I had an infection, the hospital protocol was to keep the baby in the NICU and give him antibiotics. Nobody told me they would give him formula. Nobody asked my permission either. They acted like it was a life and death situation that he eat immediately and just fed him Similac.

"If I would have known that the little amount of milk I had (which was actually normal) was considered insufficient for a baby receiving antibiotics, I would have investigated a breast milk bank so he could get real breast milk immediately instead of formula. Because he was a C-section baby and got antibiotics, his intestinal lining was not seeded with "good" bacteria. All the internal flora was screwed up with antibiotics, so we had to fight his colitis and these terrible bloody, mucus-y, green stools. I was a frightened new mom with a baby screaming from tummy pain. It was awful." —Inna S.

If being prepared and thinking through all possible scenarios makes you feel more comfortable and in control, you may want to ask about the NICU protocol at your hospital. If the thought of the NICU scares you or stresses you out, then feel free to let it go. Most babies are born full-term, free of immediate medical issues and never spend any time in the NICU.

Expectations &
A Bad Hospital Experience

The reality of a Postpartum Recovery floor is not what TV episodes are made of. Everywhere you turn, there's blood, urine and breastmilk, not to mention crying day and night. Sometimes from the babies, too.

Hopefully, this topic will be so irrelevant to you that you will make fun of me for even bringing it up (i.e., "I don't know *what* this chick was talking about–a *bad* hospital stay? Room service, Wi-Fi and a flat-screen around every corner... it put the Hilton to shame!"). If that's your story, that is awesome and I am truly happy for you. Feel free to go right on to the next topic.

Okay, now that it's just those of us who can relate, please know that you are not alone on this. Many delivering moms–first time and beyond–have bad, really bad or simply craptastic birth and postpartum experiences in the hospital.

Would it be better at home or a birth center? I've never experienced either so I can't say. Giving birth in a hospital was essential to my husband and me for several unwavering reasons. Nonetheless, after delivering at three different medical centers in three different cities, I will say the quality and style of perinatal care can vary widely by location.

Recently, a neonatologist friend remarked that whenever expectant couples are given a hospital tour, they see only the Labor & Delivery floor, not Postpartum Recovery. Why? Well, patient privacy, cleanliness, containing potential illness and a general lack of camera-ready L&D excitement are all factors. However, the reality of Postpartum Recovery is not pretty. There's non-stop blood, urine and breastmilk, not to mention crying all day and night–sometimes from the babies, too.

Bottom line, if in the 48 hours after giving birth you find yourself itchy, hot, cold, sweaty and uncomfortable, if you can't sleep because of plastic mattresses, glowing lights and ceaseless beeping, or if the "Postpartum Parade" is really getting you down, and you find yourself *hating* the hospital and wanting, wishing, begging to just go home, I'm so sorry. I can relate and it's the pits. And if the discomfort, annoyances and irritation of those 48 hours leave you with a sour taste about early motherhood, you're not alone.

Many new moms say they wish they'd known they didn't have to be "happy" every moment following birth, and that feeling upset didn't mean they weren't grateful for their babies. Moms can love their babies and feel like crud at the same time. Yet another shining example of exceptional maternal multi-tasking.

It would have been a relief to have permission to say that postpartum recovery stinks and it's a gigantic pain to feel like crud while trying to learn how to breastfeed and care for your baby.

Fortunately, you and your daughter or son have tons and tons of memories to make together. While the birth and welcoming of a new baby is a landmark life event, the 48 hours in recovery do not define a mother-child (or father-child) relationship. Those post-birth days more closely resemble a spluttering start to one's physical and emotional recoveries from pregnancy and birth, not an encapsulation of familyhood.

Furthermore, if you leave the hospital unable to even look anyone in the eye because you're so ticked about something someone said, or how many people interrupted your tiny windows of sleep, or because the lactation consultants or nurses were driving you crazy, and you wish you could forget the whole thing and you're terribly disappointed that these experiences are now part of your memories of your baby's birth, it's okay. You're not alone here either. Lots of other women have felt that way and the feelings soften with time.

Someday (many months or years from now) it may make a good story. I have told my oldest (now 8 years old) bits and pieces of the monkey show that was my two-day, post-birth hospital stay with him—just the light stuff, of course—and it's truly therapeutic to laugh about it together. It took about four years for me to see the humor, but now those 48 hours are just one experience with him out of so many. It didn't define our relationship or me as a mother. It was just super-duper craptastic.

What Not to Wear

Okay, this is not an advice book, but I'm just going to say it: *Whatever you do, do NOT try to wear your pre-pregnancy clothes (especially your jeans) home from the hospital!* Many, many women (myself included) still look eight months pregnant for a good long while after giving birth. I had heard the saying, "Nine months on, nine months off," but it didn't really sink in that I would be wearing maternity clothes for at least two months after delivery until with my own eyes I saw my puffy, deflated belly flapping in the breeze.

After my first birth, I wore workout pants for the first three months, and by the time I got to my third birth, I was strictly in elastic waistbands until at least month five. Pants with buttons and zippers remained in hibernation until about eight months postpartum, but they did eventually re-emerge. In fact, the combination of exclusive breastfeeding and carrying two children up and down the stairs several times each day siphoned off all the baby weight and then some by my third child's first birthday.

Go easy on yourself here, Mama. Getting dressed during postpartum can be daunting, dreadful and demoralizing. For the foreseeable future a good postpartum fashion mantra may be, "I just had a baby and I look great… I just had a baby and I look great…" Repeat as needed. It is 100% true. You did just have a baby and no matter how floppy you feel (I'm right there with you, by the way), _you do look great!!!_

Your Lovely Parting Gifts

We live in a pretty "freebie-oriented" culture, but just in case you didn't know…

"Take everything in the isolette (the little bed/cart on wheels). Not the mattress and stuff like that, but seriously, everything else. Take it. Lord knows you paid for it. Your isolette will be stocked with diapers, premade tiny bottles of formula (shelf-stable), alcohol wipes, petroleum jelly—the works. Take it home with you.

"Even if you plan to exclusively breastfeed, you will feel such a sense of relief knowing if something goes awry at 3 a.m., you already have a teeny bottle of formula ready-made in your hospital swag bag."—Tracey B.

Not Wanting to Go Home

We've already discussed the feelings of hating the hospital, feeling hot, exposed, uncomfortable and being really sick of putting on a happy face for the staff. Many new mothers have these kinds of feelings. But what if you don't feel like that? What if you really *don't* want to go home?

What if taking care of your baby without the nurses seems overwhelming? What if your baby has been in the NICU and the nurses have been doing the lion's share of the baby care? What if you don't really feel comfortable with the medicine regimen, or even feel competent to breastfeed?

If that's how you feel, please know you are not alone. Many new parents have those feelings and worries, and *with support things will get better.* There are so many people that *want* to help you and your baby. You may be surprised how many people you have in your life who are there for you, no matter what. And even if you feel you don't have anyone, there are so many folks outside your circle of family and friends who *do* understand and want to help you and your new family get on steady footing at this transitional time. Reach out and talk to us—we *want* to be there for you. Your willingness to connect amidst all the new mama craziness is amazing!!!

You can call our Warmline 941-301-8819 and leave a message (Monday-Thursday messages are returned within 24 hours, Friday messages are returned the following Monday), connect with us on Facebook www.facebook.com/postpartumsupportflorida, or visit our website www.postpartumflorida.org and contact us via email. Or if you're outside Florida, visit www.postpartum.net for resources and support in your area. We are moms who've experienced tough stuff postpartum and are here to support other new moms (and dads) as they adjust to parenthood and all the ups and downs that come with it.

CHAPTER 5

POSTPARTUM ADJUSTMENT

It Just Got Real

"I knew the postpartum period would not be glamorous, but I had no effing idea. I knew I'd be crazy, but again, no effing idea. I don't think there's any way to really prepare for it other than to know it's a hell of a ride, and there are a few things that might help, or mean you need some help."
—Angie G.

So now you're home, and if everything feels unstable and shifty at the moment, that's because it is. If you try to understand it, question it or worry about it too much, it may only scare you. You are now in the postpartum phase, outside of hospital recovery, removed from the birth experience, but still in a "Fourth Trimester" with your baby. For the next few months your baby still needs your body, your touch, your smell and your sounds as something of a shield against the harsh and relentless stimuli of his/her new environment.

Whether you want to talk about your feelings, write about them (chat boards and Facebook pages are great venting spots) or wave your anxieties away, many new moms look back at early postpartum and agree that you can't really understand the massive feelings and changes in the days (and weeks and months) after birth. Similar to adolescence, it just starts and you do your best to hang on without losing your grip, but know this—you are not flying solo, Mama. There are lots of us clinging to the rear bumper of motherhood right along with you, and we're all in this together.

Redefining Power & Control

When mom brings baby home, she may feel a seismic shift in the world she once (mostly) controlled, felt free in and understood. After birth, everything changes so quickly, she can feel completely overwhelmed and powerless. To stabilize and move forward, she may need to temporarily redefine "power" and "control," so she doesn't feel emotionally and mentally flattened.

When a baby comes home, everything changes, and for a while things may feel somewhat (or totally) out of control. But please know this... *you still have power and control, just in a different form.* Each of us has the power to be kind to ourselves, to nourish ourselves with good thoughts such as, 'I am a good person. I don't have to be 'perfect' to be good,' and 'This is really hard, and it will get easier. I am working really, really hard and doing a good job.' And you are.

As new mothers, even though everything can feel out of control at times, we do have power and control in our worlds–the power to control ourselves. And if we don't feel able to control ourselves, we still have the power to reach out for help to find a new sense of control and empowerment. As we say to our kids when they're in school, "You can only control yourself. We can do our best not to let others' behavior and moods control you."

Even as a perfect storm of exhaustion, isolation and upheaval rages around us, and threatens to invade our hearts and minds, we still have power and control–the power to listen to and trust our instincts, draw boundaries and counter self-destructive inner monologues with positive thoughts and actions, and reach out for the support we need. There are so many women who understand and are there for new moms as they transition, whatever the situation. Get in touch with us at www.postpartumflorida.org or www.postpartum.net anytime. There's safety in numbers, Mama. You do not need to go through this transition alone.

Getting "Back to Normal"

"My postpartum period with my daughter is a total blur. I hardly remember anything about her first year. I guess that's nature's way of ensuring the propagation of the species. If we remembered how much a lot of this sucks, we wouldn't keep going back for more!"–Selma G.

Once you and baby are home, you may be anxious to get back to normal. Normal you, normal partner. Sure, you know the sleeping thing is going to be tough for a while, but everything else? It really shouldn't be *that* shaken up. After all, you only brought home a baby. People do that every day in every country in the world, so what's the big deal, right? *Right?* I'm just going to get back to *normal. Normal, dammit!!! NORMAL!!!!! AHHHHHH!!!!!!!*

It was healthy to get that out. Yes, the desire to "get back to normal," whether it's following the birth of your first, second or tenth child, is very, well, *normal.* We often don't realize how drastically something is about to change, or has changed, until well after the fact. Then, there's no road back, only forward. Time to find a "New Normal."

Taking Care of You

So, you and I have now weathered some pretty huge moments together, so are you willing to do something, even if it's just to humor me? Will you please consider letting go of any latent beliefs that it's somehow indulgent or self-centered to prioritize taking care of yourself? Feel free to write a note to this effect, and tape it to your baby's changing table, where you can read it routinely. I found out the hard way that putting yourself dead last is a recipe for disaster, and am now a true believer in the power of inexpensive, yet effective, Take-Care-of-Mom techniques such as vertical hydrotherapy and boxed multi-meal solutions. (Also known as "showers" and "cereal," respectively).

Hopefully, others are available to take care of you at this time, too. Some new moms employ postpartum doulas, and appreciate their wrap-around style of support (visit www.dona.org to find a certified doula near you). If a doula isn't an option, and you don't have others to help you during your postpartum recovery (many women don't–grandmothers who can't be present, husbands who work all the time, stress in the family and more), *you have got to be in charge of taking care of you first. You, as the mother, are the bedrock of the family, and **when you take care of yourself, you are taking care of your baby and family, too.*** In early motherhood, there are some corners you can cut, and some you can't, but *YOU* are never a corner to be cut, Mama. You are the center of the whole operation.

I don't mean to sound bossy, I only aim to plant a seed of permission so when you are home with baby and 10 free minutes appear, and you can choose to either fold the laundry or watch something funny on TV and eat with two hands, I hope you'll allow yourself to take a break *without feeling guilty*. Mothers at home with little ones need lots of breaks, even teeny breaks—no babysitters required. For example, going into a different room for a little while and reading, or sitting on the front step breathing deeply for five minutes. If you recall, folks in the workplace take lots of breaks—big and small—and have people to talk to. Just because you're home does *not* mean you have any free time. A mom has to choose to take those momentary breaks for herself, for her own sanity.

Expectations & "Enjoying the Baby"

"In my humble opinion, the first three months have some sweet moments, but overall they are the total pits. Just remember, there're not predictive of the future. They're the uphill part of the postpartum marathon. They aren't the 'Motherhood Experience.' There are lots of times that it's more than okay to just put your head down and get through it."—Raina C.

Oh Lord, expectations. We all have them, and they can really screw with our heads. The expectations we have of ourselves as mothers, our partners as fathers, our babies and all our dearest maternal fantasies can be a lot to face, and even more to let go of. Often our expectations of motherhood revolve around how well (we believe) we will understand our babies. We also may have expectations of ourselves to be "perfect" mothers–endlessly calm, energetic and patient. We may have had this type of mother-figure in our lives, or we may have only imagined such a person based on women we knew or works of fiction, but the origin of our expectations matter less than simply understanding these are dreams and images only. They may inspire us or make us feel like failures, but these expectations are not a reasonable measuring stick of whether we are "good mothers."

Another common expectation of motherhood is that we, as mothers, will "enjoy the baby." Right. After we've been torn from stem to stern, are adjusting to status as a food source and the accompanying razor-blade gums, not to mention coping with levels of sleep deprivation that would make grown men cry. You may, in fact, have film footage to illustrate this point.

What does "enjoy the baby" even mean? Enjoy the overall experience? Enjoy every minute? That's, as my 5-year-old says, "Totally nutso-banana cakes." People say "Enjoy the baby" because they *wish* they had enjoyed their babies, not because it's actually *possible to* enjoy newbornhood, or even early motherhood. Enjoying sweet moments and taking some video may be as good as it gets. Much of raising little children is hard and repetitive work. That's why the good Lord made them so cute.

One mother of two put it this way:

"Enjoy the baby. Duh, right? Except nothing about parenting, not from the first minute, will be exactly what you want or expect. And at some point, especially if you are crazy with postpartum hormones (and I guarantee you will be looney, it goes with the territory), you will fixate on whatever those little imperfect things are, and they will take over your life.

"If you remind yourself that it's about the baby, and enjoying those precious, brief moments of newbornhood, some of that noise will fade into the background. I know it's not the same for everyone. So much of my daughter's early newbornhood was exactly the opposite of what I imagined, and the only thing that got me through was reminding myself to enjoy the baby. I would repeat it to myself over and over, like a mantra."–Angie G.

Maternity Leave

Maternity leave will not be a break. You will not get the chance to catch up on projects at home. You will not have "free time."

The reality of maternity leave tends to be a cruel joke. A mom of two captured the essence:

"Maternity leave will not be a break. You will not get the chance to catch up on projects at home. You will not have 'free time.' I thought I'd have loads of free time. I laugh hysterically at my naive self. Maybe someone else could have swung it. I considered myself a gold-star mama when I got a shower that didn't somehow involve me running across the bedroom, dripping wet, to soothe the baby."–Angie G.

And several moms agreed:

"Just accept that you will be constantly exhausted at least in the first six weeks, if not the first six months, when the sleep starts to stretch out at night. Do NOT try to 'catch up' on scrapbooking, basement cleaning, that book you were writing or any other big projects during your maternity leave (which is also 'the 4th trimester'—birth to three months). You are still nurturing this growing life every bit as much as when you were pregnant, except now you've added crying, lactating and never having free hands to the mix. That is your only project. We all wish we had known to expect nothing more from maternity leave than simple survival. Period."—Annie T., Angie G. & Sarita C.

More On New Dads

Get Dad involved early and often. Even if he doesn't do things they way the books (or you) say, it's a huge bonus for everyone.

Now that you're home, this is where the rubber meets the road. Habits and practices will start to get set, and while a lot of moms feel the need to "protect" their partners from the insanity of newborn care, or feel inexplicably impatient with them for not "doing things right," getting Dad involved early and often is a huge bonus for everyone.

The more Dad interacts with baby, the more his confidence grows, the more breaks you have, the better baby and dad's relationship becomes. This is especially valuable when toddlerhood hits and everyone's patience gets stretched. Many new moms say if they had it to do over again, they would have made more of an effort to let Dad in, let him try, and let him (within reason) fail. After months of parenting, these moms see it's okay for parents to make mistakes. That's how we learn.

Looking Eight Months Pregnant With a Newborn

Most women say they know in their minds it takes time to lose the baby weight, but abstract knowledge doesn't make us any less uncomfortable or impatient with ourselves. The truth is, it's often nine months on and nine months off—or more. Your body is still in shock and recovering from pregnancy and birth, and it will be that way for a while. You just spent nine months gestating a new human life, for heaven's sake, there is bound to be some fallout—a term that also may describe the condition of your hair and your boobs at this point.

Not to worry—there are *many moms who* are in the same boat as you right now. While many of them put pressure on themselves to get back to pre-baby shape ASAP, it doesn't necessarily make it happen that much faster. Feel free to put those jeans on the highest closet shelf, (or better yet, have your husband/partner hide them from you), and don't even entertain the thought of trying them on until *at least* six months postpartum, and more like nine to 12 months, for many.

The ugly truth is post-birth physical recovery takes time and can be frustrating. For some women, the whole experience took a toll on their self-esteem and enjoyment of early motherhood, and wish someone had told them they would still look pregnant long after they delivered. One mom said if she had it to do over again she would:

"... keep a better sense of humor about what a train wreck a woman's body can be for a while after delivery. It isn't going to last forever, and breastfeeding alone burns a ton of calories. You just may not see the effects for several months because your body is adjusting to the new role of being a non-pregnant food source. I should have cut myself some slack, for God's sake. I mean, it's one year out of my whole life."
–Marita D.

Speaking for myself, quite honestly, I always hate how I look in the first three months postpartum, as I am not one of those women who "snaps back." I don't even like to take any pictures as a family during that time because *they* all look so cute, whereas I look fresh from Three Mile Island.

If it takes you more time to resemble yourself–body, hair, skin, coherence–than it seems to take others, you are not alone. It may take longer than you expected/hoped, but it'll happen. One thing to bear in mind, however… things may not be exactly where you left them, so to speak, as gravity begins to take its toll. As one mom said, *"I'm not sure what's become of my tush, but my collar bone has never looked better."*

Stitches, Coughing & Laughing

"With every cough I became more afraid that I was going to split my stitches and end up right back in the hospital like a stuck pig. I was totally freaking out."—Inira V.

If you end up with stitches, whether across your belly or "framing the old hoo-haw," as one second-time mom eloquently put it, coughing and laughing in the first week post-birth is going to hurt. With all the advice, papers and general harassment so many new moms endure upon discharge and via the Internet, a critical mass of women have remarked that they wish someone had warned them before going home that any sneezing, laughing and/or especially coughing with their new stitches would be not only painful, but a bit terrifying.

Why terrifying? Here's what new mom Inira said:

"I picked up some kind of bizarre virus or something in the hospital and within 48 hours after discharge I started to cough uncontrollably for a few minutes every hour or so. It was awful on so many levels—trying to keep baby latched on, worrying that I'm passing on some mystery illness and then feeling like I'm splitting my stitches from my episiotomy every time I had to cough, which I could not stop doing!

"Every time the coughing spells came up, the stress on my stitches hurt so much I teared up. I was totally terrified that I was going to split my stitches and end up back in the hospital bleeding like a stuck pig, and I wouldn't be able to nurse my baby because I knew if I was admitted as an adult patient, they wouldn't allow me to keep a minor in my room, nor would they admit him as a pediatric patient. I was totally freaking out.

"*Finally, a friend of mine who happened to be over saw the kind of pain I was in. She had me sit on a towel, and pull it up between my legs whenever the coughing came on to keep pressure on the stitches. It did help some, as did her reassurances, but I was still so upset. It was painful and it was scary, and no one said anything about it upon discharge.*

"*It only makes sense to me to tell postpartum patients, 'If you have perineal stitches, sit on a towel and pull up (in other words, apply pressure) if you have to sneeze or cough (or laugh, though you may not be laughing about jack at this stage), and if you have abdominal stitches, hug a pillow or something to your lower belly. It will help.' New moms need some instructions on how to cope with and care for their stitches. I was just lucky I had a friend over. A lot of women don't have anyone to help them through the post-birth stuff.*"–Inira V.

More on Breastfeeding

"*Breastfeeding was way more frustrating than I ever thought it would be. Thank God for a good lactation consultant. I was ready to give up as a complete failure the 2nd night home when I just couldn't get him to eat and all he would do is scream until he was hoarse. He finally started latching without a breast shield, but man, my nipples hurt.*"–Diana B.

You're now probably somewhere between Day 3 and 23 of Breastfeeding, and you may be finding that it takes a while to get the hang of it. That's not the whole truth. You may be finding it's so painful you could die (see Chapter 3: The First Breastfeeding Latch for more). Your baby may be latching on fine, and you're starting to produce milk, but you are so engorged you feel like your breasts are going to explode, and latching on hurts like no stinking book ever expressed. "Slight discomfort," they said. Are you kidding me?

Is this nonsense about "slight discomfort" propagated because alleged "experts" and providers believe if women know how excruciating early breastfeeding can be, they wouldn't do it? I think we're tough enough to take the unvarnished truth.

It's not uncommon during this stage of breastfeeding adjustment for moms to sometimes feel scared or upset when baby starts crying to be fed. Moms know they have to get baby on the breast again, their nipples haven't toughened up yet and baby's little gums feel like little razor-sharp pliers. In fact, one mother said:

"When my husband asked what it feels like when the baby latches on, I politely suggested he go fetch a vice grip from his tool box and affix it to his &$#*. It actually may have been more hostile than polite, come to think of it, but he didn't ask again, and he was Johnny-on-the-spot with the Lanolin after that. 'What does it feel like?' Do you really want to know?"–Natalie K.

For the first 3-5 days postpartum, it may seem like nothing is happening breastfeeding-wise, but most moms feel their milk come in somewhere around Day 5. After that, latching may be painful for a couple of weeks or so. As the other books say, don't wash your nipples with soap, take warm showers and express milk to help with engorgement, use lanolin and/or wool nursing pads to protect your nipples and consider taking a bath towel to bed with you the first few weeks. (Often your milk comes in and leaks all over you the moment, or moment before, baby cries out. No joke.)

If you get mastitis, you will need a prescription for an antibiotic to get well. You should start feeling better about 12 hours after the first dose, but in the meantime it's like you've been hit by a train, so start taking it ASAP.

It can take a while to get the hang of breastfeeding, and that includes getting your nipples adjusted to the baby's latch and sucking, but it gets easier and after 3-4 weeks it won't hurt anymore. It may actually feel relaxing. You'll probably still feel the needle-like prickles of your milk coming in and letting down which some women find strange, but the latching will likely be nothing.

If breastfeeding still hurts, starts to hurt again and/or you feel a lump in your breast, you could have a clogged duct or mastitis. Mastitis is a breast infection and is marked by a high fever, red streaking and/or a hot spot(s) on the breast. This is serious and nothing to mess around with—so call your doctor's office as soon as possible. If it is mastitis, you will need a prescription for an antibiotic to recover. You should start feeling better about 12 hours after the first dose, but in the meantime it's like you've been hit by a train, so you'll want to start taking it ASAP.

Still Bleeding

Yep, you will be bleeding for up to a month following birth, though hopefully you have downgraded (or upgraded, depending on your perspective) from the crazy cheesecloth/mattress day to XL dollar bin underwear and super plus maximum strength maxis. But nonetheless, you are still bleeding. After not having your period for nine months, you may find this a total pain in the neck. Or lower. Many women are shocked at how heavily they bleed, and for how long. Personally, I felt disgusting, but finding time to take a shower was... well, as I mentioned earlier, I flunked vertical hydrotherapy my first time around with motherhood, but I am now wiser. And more fragrant.

Again with the Bathroom Issues

Just checking in to see how you're doing on this one. Hopefully you do not have the soreness-episiotomy-constipation trifecta going on, but if you do, just remember what many new moms wish they'd known—whether from a provider or a book or an email update—*to keep taking Colace at home and eat flaxseed and yogurt.*

"Take Colace. Take a lot of it. Take it for at least six weeks postpartum. Longer doesn't hurt. Taking it not long enough will. I promise."–Tracey B.

Lastly, please remember, if you can only go No. 1 (or 2) in the shower for a while, that is perfectly acceptable. What happens in the bathroom stays in the bathroom. Until potty-training, that is.

"Sleep When the Baby Sleeps"

Feel free to strangle anyone who suggests this. Seriously, it's a good idea in theory, and some can do it, but if you have other children at home, or you just can't fall asleep on cue, you don't have to stress yourself out. Instead, you can use the time to do something relaxing for yourself–take a shower, eat a meal in peace, "de-pile" the house, visit us at www.facebook.com/postpartumsupportflorida www.postpartumflorida.org, www.postpartum.net, or, as my aunt says, *"Sit in a corner and drool."*

Seriously, though... while it is unreasonable and downright annoying to feel pressured to sleep every time the baby sleeps, (WARNING: Advice pending) *protecting your sleep is of the utmost importance. Without sleep you will not feel well (read, "crazy").* In fact, eventually you will get so used to being sleep-deprived, you won't even know you are exhausted. That's when things can get really messed up. *Consistently having trouble sleeping, even when the baby sleeps*, or staying awake between night feedings to write thank you notes or Christmas cards, *are red flags of potential Postpartum Distress.*

The one best thing you can do to support your physical and mental health is to *protect your sleep*. Now, hold on... before you get annoyed at me for saying that, believe me, I get it. I did not sleep more than one or two hours at a time after my first and fourth babies were born for months and it nearly sent me around the bend. Getting sleep while caring for a newborn can be *extremely* challenging. That's why everyone says "sleep when the baby sleeps," right? Uh-huh.

Yet, for some women this strategy just intensifies their already deepening sense of confinement. If they sleep when their babies sleep, they never have any time alone to regroup, listen to silence, or simply concentrate. For that matter, if mom drops everything to sleep, who's going to do the laundry, pay the bills, and do the shopping? And when does a person eat, shower, or go to the bathroom? What if mom has older children to care for? Or has to go back to work outside the home? I don't know, Mama. I wish I had some satisfying answers.

It's not right or healthy that so many women have to shoulder so much alone. Still, the truth is *you are recovering from growing and pushing another human being out of your body, whom you now are caring for around the clock. Please consider grabbing sleep anytime you can and do not feel guilty about it. It's just a few weeks or months out of your whole life.* If it helps, you can reframe the issue and imagine you are recovering from a major operation or the flu, and you have to sleep to get your strength back.

Incidentally, I don't know why more physicians don't tell their postpartum patients to sleep as much as possible in the first three months post-birth. In many other cultures postpartum mothers aren't even allowed out of bed for weeks or months. Clearly, other societies recognize that sleep isn't a bonus, sleep is as vital to wellness as nutrition and breathing, and we need to do better giving our new moms permission and encouragement to *prioritize and protect their sleep in the postpartum period.*

If you are not able to sleep, please reach out to www.postpartumflorida.org or www.postpartum.net for the resources you need so you can get some rest and prevent things from going downhill fast.

More on Older Children, Visitors & Feeling Judged

This is your recovery from birth. You have permission to do what you need to in order to take care of yourself so you are well and able to care of your baby. And if that means no visitors, then by all means, no visitors, no questions asked.

It may come as a really crummy surprise to you that all the people you thought you'd be excited to share this beautiful experience with are not what the doctor ordered. At. All. Whether it's your children, your friends, your family or even your partner, you may feel like being left, in one mother's frank description, *"the eff alone"* with your baby, or even just *"the eff alone"* period.

When you consider all you've experienced throughout pregnancy, labor, delivery and early postpartum, not to mention the conception period (as that can bring its own stresses for many couples), you may need, as the same mom said, *"Some Goddamn space!"* You can likely gather the raw, honest perspective she generously offered me, and she makes a powerful point–personal space is key to recharging and regaining some energy and balance following birth.

Some moms wish someone had told them they might *not* want to have a bunch of people around soon after birth (as in, a couple months), and if they change their minds about having visitors, whether at home or at the hospital, *that is okay.* In fact, *this is your recovery from birth, and you have license do whatever you need to do to take care of you, so you are well and able to take care of your baby.*

Many women have shared how guilty and conflicted they tend to feel about wanting or not wanting to spend time with their older children after a new baby comes. On one hand, a mom may be anxious to "put in some quality time" with her older children after being away in the hospital for a couple days (or more), but after taking the big kids to the science museum or the zoo, mom may feel completely exhausted, irritable and frustrated that she couldn't make the outing work "the way it used to."

"Anyone going from one to two kids, take note—there is a big adjustment period that is not so much on the kids' part, and it can really sucker punch you."—Angie G.

For some moms, it's difficult to face how the addition of a new baby will change what was a fairly settled family dynamic. A dynamic that may not have been perfect, but was familiar, comfortable and (somewhat) predictable. When baby comes home, it may feel as if everything is up in the air. Not only is mom getting to know her new baby, she may also be feeling hyper-sensitive to all her children's (and her partner's) growing pains. This adjustment process can feel overwhelming and extremely stressful.

If you have had it up to your eyes with the caravan of well-meaning (or not so well-meaning) people traipsing through your home or hospital room, you are not being "difficult," "controlling," or "selfish." You are being honest with yourself, which is actually quite admirable and increasingly a lost art.

Being honest about your needs during your postpartum adjustment is critical to your and your baby's wellness. This is where the "listening to your inner self" we talked about earlier comes into play. Being honest about one's needs can be difficult for some women and feel contrary to their self-sufficient personalities. Sometimes needing *anything* from *anyone* makes a woman feel selfish, demanding or terribly vulnerable. Still, the adjustment to motherhood can be a good time to experiment with letting one's guard down a little and allowing more support from others. Yet opening ourselves up to other people is complicated, isn't it?

The presence of others can breed unintentional pressure, too. New moms frequently feel the watchful, critical eyes of others—their partners, their mothers, their in-laws(!) and even their friends—judging them in the early days (or years) of motherhood. This pressure can add to a woman's postpartum stress. The truth is, when people judge you, it's more about them than it is about you. Most people organize the information they take in into boxes of approval and disapproval (a.k.a., making judgments) because they are psychologically hard-wired to do so, not because they are necessarily trying to drive you crazy — even though it may have that net effect.

Everyone—including those who deeply love you—will make judgments and draw nonsensical conclusions about your parenting choices. Their judgments do not mean you're doing anything wrong, nor is it anything you can control. Most important, it's powerful only if you give it power. *It is within your control to refuse to give other people's judgments any power over you.*

It's okay to **let go** of worrying about what others think of you, your parenting decisions and your style of hospitality in the postpartum period (or entirely, but that's another book). And let go, and let go, and let go. You have permission to let go of self-conscious anxiety every time it arises. Let it go. Breathe it out. Move on. The postpartum period is so intense, you have every right to change your feelings about having visitors and family (and their remarks) at any time, and that's understandable to any reasonable person. (By the way, if you ever come across a reasonable person, please let me know).

Now, to be fair, getting the visitors to go away will not be an issue for everyone. There are women for whom visitors will be a highlight, and sharing the birth, the coming home and/or the early days of newbornhood with friends and family will be extremely important. She will want those who matter most to her to visit, meet her new baby and be present for a portion of her experience. In fact, she will likely be offended if her friends and family do *not* come over, spend time with her and meet her new baby.

One mother of almost five said this about postpartum visitors:

"Time and time again, friends and family have wanted to come as soon as we get home, or even in the hospital. I get it—it's fun to come visit your friend and her newborn in the hospital, largely because when it's you in the hospital, there's nothing the least bit enjoyable about it (Please see Chapter 4: Older Siblings & Visitors). Similarly, I know it's 'fun' to see a brand-new little baby that's just come home. That said, this time I'm saying 'no' to visitors for at least the first two weeks. This little guy will have plenty of time to get to know everyone, and I can't wait to introduce him when I don't feel like absolute garbage.

"When I had my fourth child, the day I got home, two very excited, well-meaning friends came to bring meals and 'meet the baby' because, of course, it's really special to see a brand-new baby. However, God bless them, they stayed for almost an hour! AN HOUR!!! I still could barely sit down at that point, was trying to get my daughter to latch, was completely exhausted from not sleeping more than three hours at a time for nearly nine months, felt self-conscious that my older children were climbing the walls and was still so nauseated from the after pains that I could hardly focus on the words they were saying, much less respond appropriately.

"Honestly, 10 minutes would have been okay, and up to 20 could have been somewhat permissible, but an hour???? I still have no real clue what occurred during that visit, but I'm not going to tempt fate again, even if I have to make something up. I'm fully prepared to say I contracted rotavirus in the hospital and don't want to infect them. Love you dearly—catch up with you in two weeks (at least!)."–Marilyn T.

Another experienced mom had this advice/strategy for the visitor dilemma:

"When it comes to visitors at home, your willing scapegoat is your pediatrician. When everyone and their brother wants to manhandle your days-old baby, feel free to kick everyone out and say, 'Baby's doc says no visitors for two weeks/for x days after vaccines, etc.' The first part is true. The rest of it just maintains your sanity and keeps people and their germy kids away!"–Tracey B.

Nutrition

After the birth of my third child, I kept an open bag of chocolate chips on the kitchen counter from the third week to probably the fourth month postpartum. They only went away because the Christmas cookies started rolling in.

At some point in the first month postpartum, you realize you don't have two hands to do things anymore. You mostly don't even have one. Now those one-handed, high-protein, high-fat snacks from Chapter One really come in handy. Think nuts (chocolate covered, naturally), cheese sticks, shelled hardboiled eggs and dry breakfast cereal. Whether you are breastfeeding or not, your body needs to recover.

The food/nutrition thing can get especially complicated and bring on guilt and negative thoughts because quick sugar might be one of the only things that keeps you going and/or is a source of enjoyment right now. After the birth of my third child, I kept an open bag of chocolate chips on the kitchen counter from the third week to probably the fourth month postpartum. I figured, "If this is the worst the vices get, we're doing fine."

Burping the Baby (!!!)

This isn't really a baby care book, but please permit me to share with you one *extremely important baby-care tip* I wish someone had told *me*. *Burp the baby really, really well,* especially in the first 3-4 months. I was too timid to be diligent about it, and I'm certain *my oldest child would have slept better and stayed asleep longer if I had adequately burped him.*

You can ask your pediatrician and/or childbirth educator the best way to burp a baby. After four babies, I've found a firm pat on baby's lower back/bottom while doing a deep bounce (bend those knees!) with baby high on your chest/shoulder works well. Sometimes baby needs to burp two or three times in a row to get tummy relief, and if you feed baby and then put him/her in the car seat and s/he starts crying? Probably needs to burp. I can't say it enough... *burp the baby really well and every time* and you'll both feel better.

"Bumpy Start"/Sensitive Babies

The mom of a more sensitive newborn often feels embarrassed or apologetic that her baby is having more of a bumpy start, as well as guilty that she's not enjoying her baby as much as she expected to or as much as other new moms seem to be enjoying their babies.

This is tough stuff for everyone— tough to recover, tough to bond, tough to communicate with your partner and maybe tough to feel like things will ever get better. One mom of a "bumpy start" baby said:

"We tried every frickin' thing with Baby L–swing, swaddle, shush, gas drops, Reglan, in case he had reflux, you name it. He's just intense and gets so screamy when he's tired, which doesn't help him fall asleep. During his first two months, I spent hours every night sitting on a stability ball, bouncing him. It was the only thing that would calm him. I still use it when he gets really squirrelly tired.

"He started responding to a bouncy seat with a nice, peppy bounce so Daddy could get in on the baby-soothing action. The little guy had so much trouble figuring out when he wanted to sleep. Things got better, but it took a long time to get to a good place, for his happiness and ours."–Angie G.

"Bumpy start" babies present a unique degree of postpartum stress. In fact, having a bumpy start baby immediately puts mom (and dad) at the head of the line for postpartum support. The mom of a bumpy start baby often feels embarrassed or apologetic that her baby is more sensitive at this stage, and that (of course) she's not enjoying her baby as much as she expected to and/or other new mothers seem to be enjoying their babies, and as a consequence may be less likely to reach out for postpartum support. Such a shame, as the wonderful parents of bumpy start babies often need support the most! A normal response, but as one mom said:

"I wish someone had told me to just tell the truth about how I felt. Trying to hide my ambivalent feelings about my high-need newborn daughter in her first very, very rocky eight weeks made my transition and caring for her exponentially more stressful. Once she started sleeping a few hours at a time, and we got through the worst of it, we started to bond for real, and it made all the pretending seem really stupid. It was what it was, and that's life. We went through some serious crap together, and even though I still can't really face what happened in those first two months, if I had to do it again, it would have been better for me to be honest about what was happening so I could work through it and get some help."–Natalie K.

One mom remembered her days with her easily over-stimulated/sensitive baby very well, and recalled what eventually helped things improve:

"I finally realized he didn't like being a baby. Once he could roll over, then crawl and walk, we had so much fun together. When we were both cranky, I did a lot of 'fake it 'til you make it.' I smiled at him whether I felt like it or not, and it helped both of us feel better.

I feel for moms of intense, sensitive babies that don't want to be lying in one spot and always want to be bounced/held/looking around–it can be exhausting. You'll have such fun together when he can be more independent. What a fantastic little person you have in your arms... being a baby just isn't his (or her) style."–Gracie W.

Going Bald and Other Signs of Hagdom

"Why can't I pull myself together? So-and-so doesn't look like her hair is coming out in clumps and... yes, yes.. those are buttons on her jeans, dammit, buttons! I'm still muffin-topping over my maternity pants!"

Many of the pregnancy and "First Year" books talk casually about "hormone changes" and "your body adjusting to breastfeeding/not being pregnant," but what many new mothers wish someone had told them is that you may sort of go bald and generally look like a hag for a while after you give birth. This does not happen to everyone, which makes spreading the word all the more vital.

Frequently new moms lament that they drag themselves, engorged and balding, to a new moms group, only to find every other mom there looks amazing! *Amazing!!* Like, going-out-with-full-hair-and-make-up-amazing. Baffled, the haggish moms observe these perfected individuals with disbelief—*"How can she look so great? I have one contact in and I don't think I even brushed my teeth!"* Following their initial shock, these half-blind, gum-chewing moms' wonder then turns to discomfort and self-consciousness. *"Why can't I pull myself together? She doesn't look like her hair is coming out in clumps and... yes, yes.. those are buttons on her jeans, dammit, buttons! I'm still muffin-topping over my maternity pants!"*

(Sigh)... Postpartum recovery–it's not pretty, but you *always* are, Mama, and that's a fact. Even when you don't feel like it. *You are doing the hardest job there is–caring for a new human being*, and that alone makes you divine, marvelous, and extraordinary (plus all your other regular awesomeness, of course). As Dorothy of "The Golden Girls" once wisely said, "It's not easy being a mother. If it were, fathers would do it."

Bottom line, if you don't look at all like yourself for a while– as in "months"–after you deliver, you may kind of hate it, but it is 100% normal. I don't know how anyone could possibly *NOT* feel like the walking dead after growing, carrying, and pushing a brand new person out of her own body, and then becoming her round-the-clock food source/supplier, for heaven's sake. Please know this–a lot of stuff goes down in the first twelve months post-birth, but you will find your spring again. Just be aware, however, that like pregnancy it's a process of months, not days.

For what it's worth, we are allowed to dial down our personal expectations and let it ride through the first year. There is no perfect wife, mother or woman. You <u>are</u> amazing exactly as you are, and you will meet whatever long-term goals you have for yourself. Moreover, we have no idea what's going on in the lives of these alleged "perfect-looking people." It's a cliché, but you really can't judge a book by its cover, and what's more, a little hagdom keeps us humble.

As one mom put it:

"I looked like death warmed-over for at least two months after my son was born, and honestly, it took longer for everything to come back online with each subsequent child. However, I now accept this about myself. I can take the time to put on concealer and perfume and at least re-do my ponytail, but sometimes I just don't give a rat's a**, and that's my choice.

"At first, I thought if I didn't look like my pre-pregnant self on the same schedule as other new moms it meant I was 'behind' or wouldn't get there, but after going through the cycle a few times, I know that's not true. It just takes some of us a little longer. I'd rather have 15 more minutes of sleep or stillness than get up and do my hair and make-up to go somewhere and get spit-up, poop or breastmilk on myself. I'll start caring again next year. That's how I feel and I'm good with it."—Christina C.

The one thing is—it's overused, but true—put on your own oxygen mask first and don't feel one bit guilty about it. As one mom said:

"Keep up with self-care—fluids, vitamins, nutrition, teeth brushing, etc.:) Our Pedi said he can always tell the mother is having a hard time when she brings in an adorable, well-dressed, glowing little cutie and mom looks like she's been in a war zone. Shows that she's putting herself way last and is headed for possible burn-out."—Jane P.

It's very healthy to let things go, (sometimes we have to let things go *repeatedly*, such as disappointment over a birth experience or hurt that husband doesn't "get it," multiple times a day because holding on to hurt and disappointment only stresses us out, limits us and holds us back), but completely letting *yourself* go, a.k.a., not taking care of yourself, is not going to work. Many new mothers say they wish they'd known it was okay to do things to take care of themselves, and it doesn't mean they're being selfish, so here goes, ahem... *"It is okay to do things for yourself–that is being smart, NOT being selfish!"* Any questions?

Missing Being Pregnant

"I wish we cared as much about the Postpartum Mom as we seem to be fascinated by the Pregnant Mom-to-Be. I didn't really need doors opened for me when I was pregnant, but juggling a toddler, a stroller, three bags and a hungry newborn? Yep, now would be a great time to hold open that door."
–Natalie K.

Missing being pregnant is normal, and a lot of women feel it even if they don't admit it. In our Postpartum Support Group, some women have said they were surprised they missed being pregnant, especially those who were sick through most of their pregnancy, were on bed rest or had other complications. Why do they miss being pregnant? As one second-time mother said:

"You feel so special when you're pregnant. People ask you how you're doing, once your belly pops it looks so cute (for a while), and, of course, feeling the baby move is just the best. After I gave birth, I just felt so empty. I looked at my floppy stomach in the mirror and looked and felt awful. I missed feeling my son against me. I wore him in the sling so I could feel him. It helped a little. It was hard.

"Then once baby comes, instead of being Super Pregnant Lady, I'm just another woman with a crying baby trying to nurse in a checkout line. I wish we cared as much about the Postpartum Mom as we seem to be fascinated by the Pregnant Mom-to-Be. I didn't really need doors opened for me when I was pregnant, but juggling a toddler, a stroller, three bags, and a hungry newborn? Yep, now would be a great time to hold open that door."–Natalie K.

What You Need to Recharge

Many, many new moms feel overwhelmed and/or powerless at times (or for some, all the time) as they adjust to motherhood. Yet, it seems every magazine article on postpartum wellness says the same thing: Exercise, eat leafy greens, go on a date night… give me a break. The standard coffee table recipe for postpartum wellness falls far short of what actual mothers need. Mothers are still women—individual and unique, not some Stepford focus group, and shoving all moms into lockstep on how to (properly) relax… guess what? Not relaxing.

Some women need to order their environment to get their heads straight. Others need time alone to reflect and organize their *inner* worlds/inner selves so they can feel a sense of control and balance. Still other moms may feel trapped being at home so much in the first few months, and while many mamas are devoted to breastfeeding and won't give it up, some may feel confined by a rigid nursing schedule, lonely without friendly adults to laugh with, and generally, as one mom put it, "stuck." (Please visit www.postpartumflorida.org and click on "Personality and PPD" and "Our PPD Study" for more information on the impact of personality differences in the postpartum period).

Every mother (really, every person) needs something specific to emotionally recharge, especially under stressful circumstances. Some crave privacy, quiet, and limited interruptions. Others ache for freedom, connection, and variety. In order for a new mom to recover, care for baby and healthfully adjust to the demands of motherhood, her individual needs have to be recognized, respected and responded to. I want to emphasize that needing to relax and regroup has nothing to do with a mother's love for her baby. Everyone needs time and space to recharge in her own way. *Everyone.*

It's super-convenient if someone recharges by baking a thousand chicken breasts to freeze, or thoroughly scrubbing a highchair and carseat, or making matching handcrafted outfits for every occasion, but those preferences don't make that person a *better* mother, it just makes her transition to motherhood a little smoother. How lucky to overlap your current responsibilities with your personal interests. Other moms may dread cleaning and cooking and can't even thread a needle, but have fascinating talents and interests that just don't happen to coincide with the common demands of newborn care and early motherhood.

Every mom is specific and necessary, and when there is little to no space for her best features and qualities to be expressed in the postpartum period, she may feel self-conscious and doubt her abilities as a mom. The trick to getting through the, as one mother said, "heaviness" of postpartum adjustment is to carve out tiny spaces within your changing world where you can stay tethered to your ongoing interests, and flex your favorite parts of you as you find your new rhythm.

It's not the whole enchilada of who you are, and the bridge from pre-baby-you to mother-you may be bumpy, but the postpartum year is the boot camp of motherhood. It's tough, intense, and exhausting, but it is finite, it gets easier, and you will do it and do it well. You may not enjoy it all the time, or feel comfortable with the changes that are happening to you–postpartum is much like adolescence that way–but you can carry your uniqueness forward into motherhood, find that new normal, and create your own original new you.

Beware of "Perfect" Mothers

The quiet moms in the Mom & Baby Group or playgroup may be harder to get to know amid all the crying, but much more stable, real and worth knowing

"All that glitters is not gold," as my mother says, and any new mom who lassos you into a conversation about how well her baby is nursing, how fast she lost the weight, how long baby is sleeping through the night, how much big brother/sister just *adores* his/her baby, blah blah blah is either compensating for something and/or just took her fourth non-prescription anti-depressant of the day.

Guess what? You do not have to be her friend. You do *NOT* have to give her your number to "get the babies together"... she will only make you crazy. The quiet moms in the playgroup are harder to get to know amid all the crying, but much more stable, real and worth knowing. Many new moms say they wish they'd known you don't have to try to become close friends with any and all new moms you meet. *"Just 'cause you both have babies doesn't mean you're going to besties,"* one first-time mom said.

It's sort of like going to camp or college and trying to make friends–you end up talking to/hanging around with the people you're sitting with on the first day. Then, after a few weeks or months, you realize you actually don't feel that comfortable with them. You may choose to disentangle yourself from these friends, find new ones and even go through the process of wondering, "What's wrong with me that I didn't click with them?"

Truth? There's nothing wrong with you at all. In fact, you're awesome! You're reading, reaching out, trying to make sense of all the postpartum craziness... Hells yeah, Mama... *you're rocking this!!* It's simply that making new "mom friends" is just like camp, college and cafeterias... it takes time, and there are lots of women out there who you *will* truly click with–you just weren't sitting with them on the first day. If you keep going to different mom-and-baby gatherings and keep being yourself (even if that person seems to be constantly changing as you find your "New Normal"), you will meet women you really like and develop a lifelong bond with them. Like a hostage situation.

Death, Grief, and Postpartum Stress

Frequently new mothers who are grieving the death of a loved one or a previous pregnancy or infant loss may find themselves shocked by the intensity of their grief, and so pressed by the needs of their new baby, as well as other children and responsibilities, they have little personal/emotional space to grieve and may struggle to manage their stress.

Losing someone you love is a pain beyond words, and whether expected or unexpected, past or present, sometimes mothers are shaken when their babies' arrival triggers a new grieving period for a past loss. What's worse, it may be hard for others to accept that a mama who's felt the pain of pregnancy loss, stillbirth, infant death or child death may need time to grieve in a new way. To many folks this may look like "wallowing" or "living in the past" when "she has a baby now and *should* be happy!" Ugh. Wrong answer.

It's only natural to think about the ones you've loved and lost as you learn to love another–imagining the joys that you dreamed of having beside a little one who's no longer with you as you build memories with a new sweetheart. Love, life, and death are about as complicated as it gets, and (newsflash)… *mothers are capable of having more than one emotion at a time.* We can be mournful *and* grateful, overjoyed *and* overwhelmed all at once! Astonishing, isn't it??? Enough "shoulding" all over ourselves.

Explaining it this way may help others understand: All the precious people a mother treasures are carefully kept in her heart, and when her heart grows a new room for her new baby, the loves, dreams, and losses she's experienced may knock around against each other for a while until her heart settles down again. It's not about forgetting–a mother never forgets–it's about reordering our world, and learning to cope with grief in our new circumstances.

In addition to past losses, some of the moms in our support group suffered the loss of a loved one during their postpartum year. These moms were shocked to discover their stress and grief-coping responses were "wobblier" during the postpartum period than they would have been were they not caring for a vulnerable new baby. In fact, frequently new mothers who are grieving the death of a loved one find themselves overwhelmed by the intensity of their grief, and so pressed by the needs of their new baby, as well as other children and responsibilities, they have little personal/emotional space to grieve. This can make coping a challenge and exaggerate post-birth stress.

If you or someone you know experiences a loss or a resurfacing of grief in the postpartum period and are suffering, please know the key to coping can be as simple as *talking about it with someone you trust.* It may be difficult to find that person within your family if your family members are grieving, too, but there are places you can go for real, thoughtful support. Grief and loss groups can be a tremendous help, including online support through Facebook Groups and BabyCenter. I am so sorry for any loss you've suffered. Peer support in times of tragedy can be an incredibly powerful tool for healing. Please know you are not alone.

Your Inner Conversation

Many new mothers are caught off-guard by the doubt and worry they feel over even their earliest parenting decisions. The combination of the hormone changes, sleep deprivation and physical and emotional exhaustion can trigger an inner monologue of worry and negativity. If unchecked, this negative self-talk can devolve into a self-destructive habit of anxiety and doubt that multiplies when you're already stretched to your maximum.

Ugh... negative thoughts. They are a drag, and especially wily and destructive with new, isolated moms since conversing with a baby is a uniquely one-sided conversation. Negative thoughts wear convincing disguises, too—virtue, honor, selflessness, kindness, sympathy, achievement, pride, even martyrdom. These negative, critical thoughts can seem valid—like they're giving you good advice—but if the so-called "good advice" is riddled with those nasty "shoulds" we just discussed, inner insults and obscenities, exhaustion has shut off your internal filter and your mind is spinning free of gravity. It's not uncommon, but it sure is torture.

When negative thoughts start looping through your sleep-deprived, addled mind, you have the power to stop them, or at least slow them down. Every time one pops up, you have the power to replace it with an opposite, positive thought, even hundreds of times a day. Just because it popped into your unfiltered mind doesn't mean you need to take it in, try to understand it or believe it.

We can choose which thoughts to concentrate on like we choose which foods to eat. Even in the overwhelming fatigue of the postpartum period, what we listen to and believe in our own minds is still our choice. We can speak to ourselves with kindness and patience. We can nourish ourselves with positive, encouraging thoughts. Instead of worrying, "I can't do this," we can tell ourselves, "I *can* do this. I AM doing this. I'm just not enjoying it yet." "I am a good mother. I don't have to be 'perfect' to be good. This is really hard, and it will get easier. I am working really, really hard and doing a good job."

You can tell yourself good things over and over, hundreds of times a day—positive thinking is free and it definitely can't hurt—though during the exhausting postpartum period the required effort and concentration can be tough to muster. Yet, positive self-talk it is a powerful tool, especially if you're game to make it a habit. It requires no membership fees, expensive starter kits, or outfits to squeeze into, no shipping costs, child care, or parts to clean. Nope, this wellness technique starts right in your rocking chair because feeling happier can begin with us accepting that we *already* approve of ourselves *exactly as we are.*

We are good, and can never be anything but good. We have the free will to do dumb things, but we, in truth, are *good.* *Good* mothers, *good* people, *good* daughters, *good* wives. We can love ourselves exactly as we are because we are already so lovable—we just have to believe it. We exude good every day. Knowing it and owning our awesomeness can be the key to lifelong health and happiness. Why isn't this simple habit of positive self-talk more popular, revered, and taught to every new mama to share with her family? Easy. Because it's not a money-maker. There's no gadget to buy and throw away. No system to "sell." Just us... taking a stand against the inner bully.

Please know I struggled with talking nicely to myself *for years,* so I don't mean to say it's an easy switch, but for many people it really works. Personally, I started making the change after my fourth child to when Postpartum Anxiety came creeping. At Postpartum Florida we also use positive affirmation exercises in our Moms Support Group, as well as our volunteer trainings, and I can honestly say I have been *amazed* by the personal breakthroughs some moms have made by committing to changing their inner conversation and shutting that bully down.

Positive self-talk can turn things around, and, for some mamas, allow them to take their lives back. Quick heads-up–it takes about six weeks to switch your brain over from old "reflex" negative thoughts to new positive ones, and will require daily attention, so if you're having a hard time making the change for a while, it's okay. Those old inner bully grooves run deep, but if it's something you want to do you'll get there. It's as easy as complimenting yourself on all the good you do every day, the exceptional gifts you bring to your family and community, and how amazing you are. And you are. Period.

It's so simple we sometimes forget... if we eat crud, we feel like crud, and if we ruminate on inner insults, criticism, and regret, our hearts and minds can feel defensive, bitter, and hopeless. Entertaining ongoing negative thoughts and guilt really *is* like allowing yourself to be bullied from the inside. You wouldn't want that kind of abuse for anyone you love, including the most important person in your family... _you_. You are too good for that garbage. (*Note: If you want to talk more about this, feel free to email me anytime: sarahpostpartumfl@gmail.com*).

A Last Word About Breastfeeding

If breastfeeding is a goal of yours, you do not need to feel discouraged by the pain and fumbling of the first few weeks. By the end of the first month, it is highly likely that you won't need a leather strap to bite on anymore.

If you are breastfeeding, and your baby is one to three weeks old, you may be at the point where latching on has become incredibly painful. Many new moms wish someone had been more direct about the pain of breastfeeding, and how long it lasts. If you are a few weeks in, you are in the home stretch. By one month postpartum, breastfeeding should be (mostly) comfortable.

Not to say that all pain is normal. There are clear warning signs of problems. If you have a lump in your breast, cracking and/or bleeding nipples or simply feel that something about the way breastfeeding is going with your baby just isn't right, you can reach out right away to your hospital's lactation consultant, call your local La Leche League, or find a breastfeeding support group in your community. Furthermore, if you have red streaking on your breast, one or more hot spots on your breast, or a high fever with chills you may have mastitis, and you need to call your provider right away.

There are many things that can help a difficult breastfeeding situation, and having nursed four babies for a total of four and a half years, I can honestly say I am so glad I was able to breastfeed my children for many reasons–the bonding, the nutrition and my own physical recovery (the release of oxytocin during breastfeeding was about the only thing that relaxed me with my third child). So, if breastfeeding is a goal of yours, you do not need to feel discouraged by the pain and fumbling of the first few weeks. And look on the bright side–by the end of the first month it is almost certain that you'll no longer need a leather strap to bite on. Yeah, it's only kind of funny right now.

For some moms, however, breastfeeding is not possible, and if it doesn't work out as planned, it can be disappointing, stressful and, for some moms, devastating. Especially if the mother has associated some (or all) of her success as a mother on her ability to breastfeed. In other situations, bottle-feeding may have been planned, but the process of "drying up," dealing with others' disapproval and figuring out "how to bond with the bottle" can be a lot to manage. A first-time mother shared her struggle with breastfeeding and how she transitioned to bottle-feeding in a positive way:

"Not being able to breastfeed was one of the most difficult obstacles I had to overcome as a new mom. When I was pregnant, I had every intention to breastfeed, so much that I didn't even have any bottles before my daughter was born because I didn't think I would need them. All the childbirth education classes talk about how important the bonding is between mother and infant during breastfeeding, and I was so looking forward to that experience.

"Towards the end of my pregnancy when the colostrum didn't come in I started to get a little worried, but my OB told me that was 'normal,' that it came later for some mothers and not to worry because once the baby comes I would have plenty to feed her.

"When my daughter was finally born and first placed on my chest there is no word to describe the emotions I was feeling. I immediately tried breastfeeding but we were unsuccessful in the delivery room so the nurses told me to try again later—that this was normal to experience difficulty in the beginning. Time after time I tried feeding her during my stay in the hospital, but it seemed I did not have any breast milk or colostrum yet.

"Going to support groups was also discouraging because everyone was whipping out their breasts to nourish their children and here I was whipping out some chemically made concoction. I felt like such a failure and that everyone was judging me and my formula-fed baby."—
Rebecca L.

"Everyone kept telling me it was normal, to be patient, that it could take a week sometimes for milk to come in. I wanted to believe them, yet I was so nervous to bring her home because I didn't know how to feed her and I didn't want to give her a bottle. The disappointment I felt was overwhelming, I felt that I was already failing as a mother and I hadn't even brought her home yet. I couldn't stop thinking that I was doing something wrong, and I beat myself up over it for a long time.

"At home the inability to breastfeed continued, and I got increasingly discouraged and frustrated. I had breastfeeding consultants come to my house, I went to breastfeeding support groups, online forums, I talked to my OB, my daughter's pediatrician and everyone kept telling me to keep trying. But nothing was happening.

"Going to support groups was also discouraging because everyone was whipping out their breasts to nourish their children and here I was whipping out some chemically made concoction. I felt like such a failure and that everyone was judging my formula-fed baby and me. I even put off feeding my wailing infant a time or two until I left the 'support' groups to avoid embarrassment at not having the means to sustain her. Everyone kept saying, 'Don't give up, don't give up, keep trying.' So I didn't give up.

"I started pumping five to 10 times a day in an attempt to stimulate my milk and barely got splatters in the bottle. I clearly remember sitting on my bed in the middle of the night crying and attempting to pump my empty breast while my husband sat feeding formula to our baby next to me. I decided shortly thereafter that the attempt to breastfeed had become such a stress that it was taking too much energy and time away from my daughter.

"I stopped trying after about three months and started focusing on trying to bond with the bottle. I started talking to her while giving her the bottle, stroking her head, looking in her eyes, and I soon started to feel that bond everyone talks about when feeding your baby. When I think back on it now I don't have any regrets. I know I did what I had to do and my relationship with my beautiful daughter has never been affected by my inability to breastfeed."
—Rebecca L.

Sex. No, Seriously.

"I had a small 2nd-degree tear and that puppy didn't heal until nine weeks postpartum. Separate from that, I had zero, and I mean ZERO libido for damn close to six months. Thankfully, my husband is a patient man."—Angie G.

Another lovely Postpartum surprise for new moms (and dads)—Postpartum hormones are designed to get you focused on taking care of the baby you have, not having another one, so if your libido tanks in every possible way in the weeks (and months) after birth, please know it's normal and you're not alone. Aren't surprises fun?

I love what a friend and mother of three had to say about postpartum sex (or lack thereof):

"The last thing on earth you will want with lochia oozing from your vag, milk shooting out your nipples and a critter constantly hanging on you is to get jiggy with The Mister. Your OB is your willing scapegoat. He/She will tell you "no nookie til the first postpartum visit" which won't be for at least six weeks (maybe eight). Feel free to tell the Spousal after that appointment that OB says you need to heal for another two weeks. It happens especially with episiotomies and tears."–Tracey B.

The lack of remotely satisfying intimacy (or any intimacy) in the postpartum period can further strain the relationship of two already thoroughly exhausted people (or one thoroughly exhausted person and one person on the first person's sh*t list), but it seems to be worse if you and your partner think you are the only ones. Feel free to grab the man for this page. I'll wait.

Okay, ready? Ahem...

YOU ARE NOT THE ONLY ONES NOT HAVING SEX LIKE YOU USED TO. YOU ARE RIGHT IN THE DRY-SPELL MAINSTREAM. If both people (okay, usually the guy) can be patient, helpful and understanding, things will start heating up again a lot faster than if he's frumping and moping around, basically needing as much attention as another child.

Here's a newsflash, dads:
FRUMPY + MOPEY + NEEDY = NOT SEXY

Now check this out:
COMPLIMENTS + HOUSEWORK + BABY CARE = SEXY

I understand this formula is the higher math of monogamy, but I believe you fellas can handle it. Study, review, make flashcards if you must, but this is the one thing **new dads wish someone had told <u>them</u>.** You don't want to end up so far out in the cold that you see on the back of your wife's pajamas, "Closed for Business—please call again. Next Year."

Vacations, Weekends & Holidays

Oy. There's no easy way to break this to you, so I'm just going to say it flat out: Moms work harder on vacations, evenings, weekends, and holidays than they do any other time of the year. Most new mothers don't necessarily feel this shift right out of the blocks, but often somewhere around month 4-6 postpartum, you may realize you and baby have achieved something resembling a "routine" of feeding and sleeping, and any shift in that routine can unravel a precise and treasured formula for (everyone's) sleep. This can make travel difficult.

What used to be fun and spontaneous adventures, or even just well-planned long weekends pre-baby, are now a juggling act of what you (and/or you partner) *want* to do against what you feel you *need* to do for your baby's routine. Frequently, new moms feel a bit disappointed that "going away" with baby feels a little like, as one mom said, *Throwing yourself into a crackling fire pit just to see what happens. You know it won't be good, but you're just stupid enough to try."*

This won't be every mother's perspective, of course, but if you used to enjoy vacations, weekends and holidays as special times of fun, relaxation and time to recharge with your partner, and especially enjoyed being part of holidays, but not really "taking charge" of the holiday preparation and execution... well, times are changing. Many moms work harder during these "down times" than any other time of the day or the year. And all those wonderful holiday memories that you cherished and looked forward to creating for and/or sharing with your family... who made all that possible? Yes, indeed, likely someone's *mother*, and she worked her tail off to do it. This may be a good time to call her and say thanks. I have some laundry to do anyway... meet you back in 10.

"I Can't Stand My Husband"

Ah yes, that old chestnut. If I had a dime for every time a new mom has said (or thought) the above, this book would come with a bonus tennis bracelet just to cheer you up. Truly, despising one's husband is such a running theme in our Postpartum/Mothers of Little Ones Support Group, I don't even know where to begin. I tend to tread lightly on this topic because as much as women feel irritated with their partners, they are protective of them, too, and they are not eager to bad-mouth them only to wind up the subject of gossip or pity. That said, every mom needs to vent and know she's not alone in her feelings and struggles. Many, if not most, new moms go through periods of thinking their husbands/partners are total idiots. I don't know if this is yet another iteration of nature's birth-control methods, but I do know if you've ever felt this way, *you are definitely **not** alone!*

To be fair, postpartum is really tough on dads, too. They have no idea what's happening to their partners emotionally and physically, and they can't fix it so they often cope by shutting down. Women, on the other hand, tend to equate love with understanding, i.e. "If you loved me, you'd try to understand me." In a perfect world, that would be true, but understanding one's wife in the postpartum phase can be a tall order for a man. Can any man really relate to the female perinatal experience? Even with the best of intentions? I don't think so.

Here's what he may be able to do: He can help out with tasks and show love and concern in his own way. That said, I have also observed that *most men cannot fully understand the complexity of their wives' feelings and changes in the postpartum period, especially since exhaustion exaggerates emotions*. Remember when we were younger? The differences between teenage boys and teenage girls? Straightforward v. Complex? Once again this dichotomy rears its ugly head.

For the record, I am not trying to insult anyone. Many men have a beautiful capacity to be thoughtful, loving and have deep feelings, but postpartum is super-intense emotional stuff no matter who you are. For a new dad, just trying to keep up with his wife's deep feelings (and how quickly they change) is often challenging, confusing and frustrating. This is why *women truly need other women as they recover from birth and adjust to motherhood.*

Still, it's really lousy to despise the very person you, up until recently, were quite fond of, and attempt to adjust to parenthood amid a fog of tension. The stress of feeling misunderstood and irritated that your partner "just doesn't get it," combined with needing him *and* hating him all at once, can make a new mom feel more alone and unsupported than ever.

The good news is women actually have a lot of power to dispel family tension by taking charge of situations and working the old "fake it 'til you make it." If the feelings of conflict are really getting you down, and you can't yet fix how you feel on the inside (postpartum adjustment takes time), sometimes it works to start on the outside. By choosing to change some of our external behaviors, we can get things moving in a better direction.

Some new moms were glad to know they don't have to sort out their every feeling with their husbands, that parsing through each frustration doesn't necessarily solve anything or improve the relationship, and that *lots of couples are going through the exact same thing.* These ladies said they felt empowered knowing they could pick and choose what to share with whom, they could draw some boundaries around themselves, and keep certain things within their circle of women.

Please know, I'm not advocating concealing your true feelings or hiding anything about you or your wellness from your partner. These are simply a few ways to replace old, conflict-producing habits that aren't working with new, different habits when the monotony of daily life in early parenthood starts to grind on both of you, and small things mushroom into huge fights.

Instead of ratcheting through the insanity of life as the stay-at-home-mom of little ones (i.e., how many times you've cleaned the kitchen today, how much poop you've wiped off assorted living beings and how many bodily fluids you've been sprayed with), some of our Group moms made the deliberate choice to smile at their partners (whether they felt like it or not) when they first saw them. They actually practiced (it takes practice–these are new habits!) keeping their faces relaxed and open (eyebrows up), and a relaxed, even tone of voice. Oh, and saying, "Sweetheart" through gritted teeth unfortunately doesn't count–after all, it isn't what you say, it's how you say it… right?

You may be staring at this book right now thinking, "Are you kidding me? *Smile* at him? After the day I've had and the way he acts? He doesn't deserve it!" Hey, I totally get it. This isn't what you *should* do, it's what you *could* do. It all may sound disingenuous, or just plain ridiculous, and if you hate it, don't do it, but for some moms, changing their external behaviors helped improve everyone's moods and broke the cycle of exhausted cynicism that's so common in early parenting.

Sometimes women feel pressure to "make everyone happy" before they let themselves be happy, and then are pretty ticked when no one appreciates their efforts. And when Mom's not happy, no one's happy. Some find the best way to make everyone happ*ier* (no children or husbands are happy all the time), *is to be happy first, just within yourself, just for you.* After all, frequently the things that seem the most complicated are actually quite simple: If we want things to change, we need to, you know… change. If what we're doing isn't working, rather than repeating the pattern and expecting a different result, we can make an opposite choice and see what occurs. You might just make some magic happen, Mama!

It may take a few days to a week for everyone in the house to respond to your changes, and many moms say if you start forgetting to make those deliberate external choices, things will quickly slide, but the reality is *the mother sets the tone*. Just another example of how much power women *do* have to control their environments, even when things seem like they're in a state of chaos.

Many moms also say appreciating all the good you yourself are doing for the family, as well as the good things your partner is doing, rather than just observing what he (or you) is/are *not* doing at home, can help a woman *"not feel like choking her husband. At least not as often,"* according to one mom of two.

Bottom line? Sometimes it's more peaceful for both of you to ease up on "understanding each other," in the postpartum period. You are allowed to take a page from Grandma's Book of Wisdom and just smile, give dad the three-sentence summary of the day, confidently, yet kindly, give him a quantifiable task or two (he can learn the "Family Man" thing, it just takes time and patience...), then go call someone with two X chromosomes who gets it. You can catch up with him later over a bowl of ice cream (you could both use some fun together!), and don't worry, you'll like him again... there's just no cure for being a man.

Total Exhaustion

Nearly every new mom expects to be "tired," but few of us have any clue what total, desperate exhaustion feels like (and how we will cope or not cope) until we are eyeball-deep in it and drowning. As a new mom you can expect to be completely exhausted, and if you're not, you are fortunate, but don't talk about it too much–you will alienate all the other exhausted moms around you.

One mother said this about Postpartum Exhaustion:

"With my first baby I kept expecting to catch up on sleep and somehow feel rested during those first six weeks. I wish I had just accepted that it isn't possible and that living with exhaustion is just going to be norm for a while. Maybe others could put it better, but this was a huge thing for me."–Elena B.

One more thing related to exhaustion… this was touched on in Chapter 3: "Trying to Sleep at the Hospital," but it bears repeating… if you start having thoughts that worry or scare you, reach out for help immediately. Get a referral from your provider for a mental-health professional *who is experienced in perinatal/postpartum mental health complications*. You are likely experiencing "intrusive thoughts," a common and often terrifying symptom of Postpartum Obsessive-Compulsive Disorder (OCD).

Postpartum OCD is an expression of Postpartum Distress and is frequently triggered by exhaustion/sleep deprivation. Women who experience this symptom often fear they are "going crazy," but remember this—if you're *afraid* you're going crazy, you're probably not *actually going* crazy. If the scary thoughts seem to make sense to you and you are in the midst of making a *plan* to act on the scary thoughts, that would be different. That would be a sign of *Postpartum Psychosis, an extremely serious perinatal mental health complication that requires immediate medical attention.*

Please know this—*no matter how bad things ever seem, it is never hopeless.* All postpartum mental-health issues are highly treatable if addressed. Do not conceal your true feelings and worries. If you are having thoughts that scare you, please reach out for help immediately. You can go to www.postpartum.net and find local help from providers who understand. You are not alone, no matter how you feel. There is help. *You are not alone.*

An Identity Crisis

Some women feel a loss of themselves when they become mothers. One new mom said:

"It seemed like all the best parts of me were gone. I wasn't considerate, funny, thoughtful, interesting, intelligent, attractive or even nice. I tried to be those things, but I felt like I was running on ice. I couldn't even think.

"I was in so much pain post-birth, but it seemed like I was supposed to be happy, and I didn't want to be a downer, so I just pretended everything was great. It was truly exhausting, and frightening, too. I felt so alone—like I had a terrible secret and didn't know how long I could keep up the charade of pretending to be my former self.

"What's worse, I was sure once everyone in my life found out how inept I was, they'd turn away from me. I felt that after all these great expectations people had of me being a good person and good mother, I was going to let everybody down." –Laura W.

Some new moms are shocked to find that they feel a loss of their own identities when they become mothers. Whether it's because a woman is no longer at work and spending time with friends like she used to, or because she is thrust into a new peer group of "mommies"—with whom she may or may not have anything in common aside from having babies—it can be pretty tough to take on this new role of "mom" and try to shove yourself into some foreign idea of what that means. It takes time to find that new sense of self. If you're having a hard time with this, it's not just you, and it does get better.

Feeling a loss of identity can be a sign of Postpartum Distress. Many new moms experiencing identity loss or confusion have found a lot of comfort and encouragement in postpartum/new-mom-peer-support groups. You can reach out and contact www.postpartumflorida.org, www.postpartum.net or other local postpartum-peer-support resources in your area. To quote one mom from one of our Support groups, "What a difference venting and some conversation with other understanding women can make!"

Postpartum Stress & Distress

"What kicked me this time around was L's intensity first and foremost, and that led me to not having any time to spend with my two-year-old. I was so incredibly resentful of him because he took me away from my daughter. Finally, I got on board with a great therapist—rather later than I should have—and things got better.

"Objectively, life is easier now because the little man is mellowing out slowly, but surely. We also build in one-on-one time for the girl and me, even if Baby L screams his head off the whole time. Having a paid professional for me to talk to has been super helpful, too."—Angie G.

Rarely does a woman plan on having Postpartum Distress (Depression, Anxiety, OCD, etc.), but it is the most common complication of childbirth, affecting up to one out of every three new mothers. Moms who experience Postpartum Distress often say they wish they'd known how to identify it in themselves, how common it actually is and how many resources there are for help.

Over the last eight years as a mother, friend and Peer Support Group facilitator, I've observed a pattern of "shock-fear-stress-distress" among new moms. The initial shock of an unexpected issue leads to fear (because the issue is new, we don't fully understand it, and we are afraid of what we don't understand). Then, in a state of fear (which is when we make our worst decisions), we react. This reaction leads to stress (because our fear-based reaction was predictably lousy), which leads to distress (because we still have a scary new problem we've just made a little worse) and the ship begins to sink. Now the postpartum mom likely feels afraid, out of control and a deep sense of failure (because "a good mother would know what to do," we unreasonably scold ourselves).

The downward spiral of "worry-fear-doubt-failure" begins, and if left uninterrupted, intensifies in an already exhausted mother's mind. Anxiety takes over unchecked, hopelessness sets in, and if unaddressed, the new mother can find herself in a mental and emotional crater known as Postpartum Distress (PPD). PPD is a broad term for Postpartum Mood and Anxiety Disorders which includes Postpartum Anxiety, Depression, Obsessive-Compulsive Disorder, Panic, and more. The above progression is just one row of dominos to PPD, but a very common one.

If you are feeling any of the following, you are not alone, and you may be experiencing one or more expressions of Postpartum Distress, including Depression and/or Anxiety:
I feel...
- scared
- angry
- out of control
- like I'm never going to feel like myself again
- like each day is a hundred hours long
- like no one understands

- like my relationship cannot survive this
- like I'm a bad mother
- like I should never have had this baby
- like every little thing gets on my nerves
- like if I could get a good night's sleep, everything would be ok
- like I have no patience for anything anymore
- like I'm going crazy
- like I will always feel like this

If you are feeling any of the above, you are not alone, it is not your fault, and with support you will be well.

Right now is the time for you to reach out for support as soon as you can, and talk and keep talking to someone you can trust—your partner, mother, friends, the pediatrician, a childbirth educator you liked, your lactation consultant, or visit www.postpartum.net, call the Postpartum Society of Florida Warmline at 941-301-8819 and/or email us at infopostpartumfl@gmail.com.

You can also visit www.postpartumflorida.org anytime to read more about Postpartum Stress and Distress, take a Postpartum Distress Screening Scale and/or get in touch with vetted community resources and peer-to-peer support. If you are outside of Florida, you can go to www.postpartum.net, the website of Postpartum Support International, one of the most established and reliable postpartum-support organizations in the world, to find local postpartum support and resources in your community.

Furthermore, if *talking* about it is difficult—and for many women it is—many postpartum support organizations have volunteers and support providers with whom you can email and/or text one on one. Postpartum Society of Florida hosts and moderates a Facebook page at www.facebook.com/postpartumsupportflorida.

Again, the key is to *talk to someone you trust*. It is normal to feel exhausted or overwhelmed at times, but it is not okay for you to be suffering with feelings or moods that frighten you, or to be struggling to care of your baby and/or yourself. Postpartum Distress is real and terrifying, but highly treatable, and you do not have to put up with that kind of torture. It is not your fault. You do not deserve to feel that way. You are a good mother to see that something is wrong, and even though the whole motherhood situation may seem hopeless, with the support you need, *you will feel better*.*

Note: If you are having thoughts about hurting yourself or your baby, get help immediately. Please see below for resources.

*Postpartum Society of Florida is a volunteer organization providing peer support. We are not mental health professionals and cannot respond in a crisis. If you or anyone you know needs immediate assistance, please use one of the following resources:

EMERGENCY: 911

SUICIDE PREVENTION HOTLINE: 1-800-273-TALK (8255)

The postpartum period is so complicated, far more complicated than many women ever could have imagined. Like snowflakes, no two postpartum experiences are alike, and it only makes sense that each woman needs a specific combination of support as she transitions to motherhood. As one first-time mom said:

"I thought becoming a mother was going to be all about taking care of 'the baby.' I had no earthly clue what it was going to do to me! Now seven years and three children later, I really get it—nine months to get to baby, and at least a year to get a new self. It is the biggest of big deals."–Laura W.

Postpartum Distress is about many, many factors. Being honest and reaching out for help can turn a tough situation around, and often faster than you think. No matter what comes up in your postpartum experience, just remember—*you are not alone.* Understanding support is always one call (or a few keystrokes) away.

Finding the "New Normal"

In all likelihood everything really will be okay, but, as many new moms wish someone had told them, there is no 'getting back to normal.' You and your partner—and your baby—will find a "new normal."

As mentioned before, your own physical, mental, and emotional recovery, and as well as your adjustment to being responsible for an innocent, defenseless little person, is going to take time and patience and a sense of humor, too. In all likelihood, everything will shake out fine. Still, the truth that many new moms wish someone had told them is there really is no "getting back to normal." You, your partner, and your baby will find a crazy, authentic, one-of-a-kind "new normal."

A last word from a mom of four, survivor of Postpartum Depression/Anxiety, and Postpartum Society of Florida SISTER Support volunteer on adjusting to motherhood:

"You are exactly the mom your baby needs. Hang in there—early motherhood can be a wild ride, but there are great women out there who get it and can relate to whatever you're going through. Be kind to yourself, you will find your way, and above all remember, dear Mama—you are not alone!"
—Barbara T.

Time to Fly

Well, amazing Mama, you've now read the secret scoop on everything that goes down from your first contraction to baby's first birthday (a.k.a., your graduation from Mommy Bootcamp). I hope you now feel ready to "expect the unexpected" as you enter one of the most beautiful, intense and indescribable periods of your life. The upside of any experience related to babies is that good, bad or ugly, it's bound to change, and though it's a steep learning curve, you'll be an outstanding mom. Just the fact that you care enough to read books about preparing for motherhood shows how devoted you are to giving yourself and your baby a good strong start.

As a matter of fact, feel free to repeatedly tell yourself what a good mother you are. Your baby can't say it (and can't even smile at you for the first couple months—tough stuff if you thrive on feedback), and your partner won't always say it even if he's thinking it (side effect of being a man), so moms need to be their own best advocates. Say it to yourself during the long, dark nights, especially from weeks three to 12, but beyond, too. "I am a good mother... I am working really hard... This will get easier... I am a good mother and we're going to be okay." And FYI—the second year of life with your child, when sleep is more settled, and you can start having adventures together is much more fun, and can be such a treasured reward after the intensity of the first.

Birthing and raising a baby is really, really hard work. The hardest work there is for the body, heart and soul, and also the most special. After my first baby was born I was blown away by the enormity of the big picture of parenthood. I'd had happy images of life as a mother, but when reality hit, it was really overwhelming to be "the mom!" Yes, parenthood is life-changing to say the least–time, energy, patience, devotion, attention, understanding... everything. But the relationships are built just one moment at a time. Raising a child is the investment that reaps rewards throughout, and far beyond, your lifetime. I wish you and yours only the best. Please get in touch anytime, and most of all–congratulations!!!

ABOUT THE AUTHOR

Sarah Workman Checcone is the founder and Executive Director of Postpartum Society of Florida (www.postpartumflorida.org), a non-profit mom-to-mom organization based in Sarasota, whose mission is to ease the transition from pregnancy to parenthood. She holds a Juris Doctor in Law degree from the University of Miami and a Bachelor of Fine Arts degree in Musical Theatre from the University of Michigan. Sarah is also a Certified Instructor of the Myers-Briggs Type Indicator® and the MMTIC®, and the owner & founder of *Translationships: Bridging Communication Gaps* Personality Consulting (www.translationships.com). Sarah loves to sing, laugh, eat delicious food someone else cooked, be outside, encourage amazing women, and hang out with her husband and four cutie kiddos.

Made in the USA
Charleston, SC
16 June 2014